AF251649

EUTECTIC MIXTURE OF LOCAL ANESTHETICS (EMLA)

A BREAKTHROUGH IN SKIN ANESTHESIA

edited by

GIDEON KOREN

Motherisk Program
The Hospital for Sick Children
Toronto, Ontario, Canada

Marcel Dekker, Inc.   **New York • Basel • Hong Kong**

Library of Congress Cataloging-in-Publication Data

Eutectic mixture of local anesthetics (EMLA) ; a breakthrough in skin
   anesthesia / edited by Gideon Koren.
       p.   cm.
     Includes bibliographical references and index.
     ISBN 0-8247-8842-7
     1. EMLA (Anesthetics)   I. Koren, Gideon
   RD86.E47E87   1995
   617.9'66—dc20   94-32073
                                                                  CIP

*The indications and recommendations detailed in the chapters of this volume
represent the ideas of the authors and do not necessarily reflect the views
of the manufacturer of EMLA. Moreover, the reader should be aware that
different regulatory agencies in different countries may have included different labeling instructions for this preparation.*

The publisher offers special discounts on this book when ordered in bulk
quantities. For more information, write to Special Sales/Professional Market-
ing at the address below.

This book is printed on acid-free paper.

Marcel Dekker, Inc.
270 Madison Ave, New York, NY, 10016

Current printing (last digit):
10 9 8 7 6 5 4 3 2 1

PRINTED IN THE UNITED STATES OF AMERICA

Preface

Attempts to anesthetize intact skin without painful injection of local anesthetics have been unsuccessful and frustrating. Generations of pediatric and adult patients have been used to the idea that it will take one pain (the injection) to overcome another pain (the skin procedure).

The technological breakthrough that led to the introduction of the Eutectic Mixture of Local Anesthetics (EMLA) has marked a new chapter in medical thinking as related to iatrogenic-procedural pain. The availability of an effective and safe preparation has changed medical practice in two ways:

1. Painful procedures (e.g., venipuncture, lumbar puncture) cannot be accepted as such anymore. Consequently, it is probable that new generations of patients will not equate such procedures with pain and anxiety.
2. Painful procedures, which often had to be performed under general anesthesia (e.g., lumbar puncture), may now be done at much lower risk and reduced financial cost.

EMLA was introduced into the European market in the early 1980s; however, it took a whole decade before millions of North American patients could benefit from it. On the positive side, this time window has allowed scores of clinical studies to be conducted in many countries, extending its indications to numerous painful procedures.

This book reflects an attempt to assemble an international team of clinician-scientists who have studied the efficacy and safety of EMLA in a variety of indications. It is hoped that this book, dedicated entirely to EMLA, will allow physicians, nurses, pharmacists, researchers, regulatory agencies, and parents to fully grasp the amazing scope of this preparation. It is likely that many more indications of EMLA will become apparent as the experience with it increases.

I wish to thank Mrs. Niki Balamatsis and the word processing staff of our Research Institute for preparing the manuscript. Special thanks to Mrs. Nancy Hale, Ms. Teresa VanWaterschoot and Ms.Tracy Green of Astra, Canada for their dedication to this project, and to Mr. Anders Tulgren of Astra, Sweden and his team for their critical review of the manuscript.

Gideon Koren

Contents

Contents

vii

Contributors

Matitiahu Berkovitch, M.D. Department of Pediatrics, Assaf Harofe Hospital, Tzrifim, Israel

Pascale Burtin, M.D. Clinical Pharmacology Unit, Robert Debré Children's Hospital, Paris, France

Flora B. de Waard-van der Spek, M.D. Subdivision of Pediatric Dermatology, University Hospital Rotterdam—Sophia, Rotterdam, The Netherlands

Judy Donsky, B.Sc. The Hospital for Sick Children, Toronto, Ontario, Canada

Chrisoula Eliopoulos, B.Sc. Division of Clinical Pharmacology and Toxicology, The Hospital for Sick Children, Toronto, Ontario, Canada

Madlen Gazarian, MBBS, FRACP Department of Clinical Pharmacology, The Hospital for Sick Children, Toronto, Ontario, Canada

Richard Hackman, M.D. Department of Clinical Pharmacology, The Hospital for Sick Children, Toronto, Ontario, Canada

Daniel S. Halperin, M.D.   Department of Pediatrics, Clinique de Pédiatrie, Hôpital Cantonal Universitaire, Geneva, Switzerland

Paul Hwang, M.D.   Department of Neurology, The Hospital for Sick Children, Toronto, Ontario, Canada

Shinya Ito, M.D.   Department of Pediatrics, The Hospital for Sick Children, Toronto, Ontario, Canada

Joseph Kapelushnik, M.D.   Department of Pediatrics, Rothschild Hospital, Haifa, Israel

Gideon Koren, M.D.   Motherisk Program, Division of Clinical Pharmacology and Toxicology, Department of Pediatrics, The Hospital for Sick Children, Toronto, Ontario, Canada

Ram Kumar, M.D.   The Hospital for Sick Children, Toronto, Ontario, Canada

Susan Davis Lethbridge, M.D.   Thalassemia Clinic, The Hospital for Sick Children, Toronto, Ontario, Canada

Laura A. Magee, M.D.   Department of Clinical Pharmacology, The Hospital for Sick Children, Toronto, Ontario, Canada

Doreen Matsui, M.D., FRCP(C)   Department of Pediatrics, Children's Hospital of Western Ontario, London, Ontario, Canada

Lennart Ohlsén, M.D.   Department of Plastic and Hand Surgery, Uppsala University, Uppsala, Sweden

Nancy Olivieri, M.D.   The Hospital for Sick Children, Toronto, Ontario, Canada

Arnold P. Oranje, M.D., Ph.D.   Subdivision of Pediatric Dermatology, University Hospital Rotterdam—Sophia, Rotterdam, The Netherlands

Izhar ul Qamar, M.D.   Department of Pediatrics, LaRabida Children's Hospital and Research Center, University of Chicago, Chicago, Illinois

Shyam Radhakrishnan, B.Sc.   The Hospital for Sick Children, Toronto, Ontario, Canada

Michael J. Rieder, M.D., Ph.D.   Departments of Pediatrics, Pharmacology, Toxicology, and Medicine, University of Western Ontario, London, Ontario, Canada

Isabelle Robieux, M.D.   Department of Clinical Pharmacology, Centro di Riferimento Oncologico—Aviano, Aviano, Italy

Donald Rosenthal, M.D., FRCP(C)   Division of Dermatology, Department of Medicine, McMaster University, Hamilton, Ontario, Canada

Graham Sher, MBB.Ch.   Division of Hematology/Oncology, The Hospital for Sick Children, Toronto, Ontario, Canada

Kathleen Shilalukey, B.Sc., MB.Ch.B.   Department of Pharmacology, University of Zambia, Lusaka, Zambia

Anna Taddio, B.Sc.   Division of Clinical Pharmacology and Toxicology, Department of Pediatrics, The Hospital for Sick Children, Toronto, Ontario, Canada

Marinette Wyss, M.D.   Department of Pediatrics, Clinique de Pediatrie, Hôpital Cantonal Universitaire, Geneva, Switzerland

1

Pharmacology of Local Anesthetics

Doreen Matsui

Children's Hospital of Western Ontario
London, Ontario, Canada

I. INTRODUCTION

Local anesthetics are drugs used clinically to block the conduction of impulses in peripheral nerves. Because both of the active components of EMLA® (lidocaine and prilocaine) are local anesthetics, it is important to consider the pharmacology of this group of agents before focusing on EMLA itself. Knowledge of these compounds is important in the understanding of their efficacy and toxicity.

II. CHEMISTRY

A typical local anesthetic consists of hydrophilic and hydrophobic groups separated by an intermediate alkyl chain. The hydrophilic portion is usually a tertiary amine, while the hydrophobic (or lipophilic) portion is generally an aromatic residue. The intervening linkage is

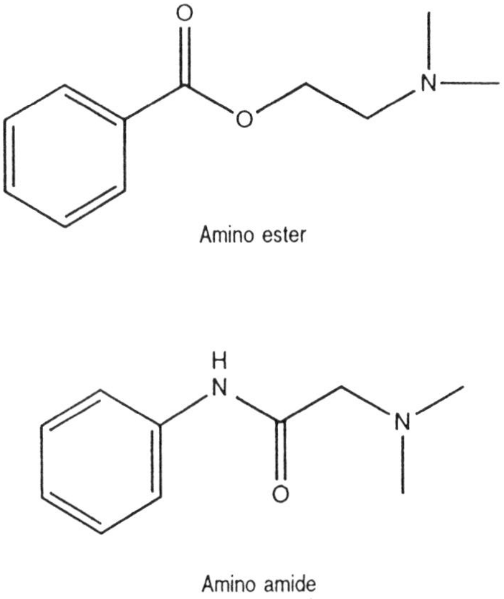

Amino ester

Amino amide

Figure 1 Two classes of local anesthetics: ester- and amide-type linkages.

either of an ester (–COO–) or amide (–NHCO–) type (see Figure 1); hence these compounds are commonly divided into two classes: the amino esters (e.g., procaine) and the amino amides (e.g., lidocaine). The nature of the ester or amide bond determines certain pharmacological properties of these agents, for example, their principal metabolic degradation pathway [1].

In general, local anesthetics are weak bases with pKa values ranging from 7.6 to 8.9 [2]. Local anesthetics exist in solution as an equilibrium mixture of unionized (free base) and ionized (cationic) forms, depending on the pH of the solution. At the pKa, 50% of the anesthetic is ionized [3]. The amide type anesthetics have lower pKa values than the esters; thus, the proportion of unionized drug present at physiological pH is greater with the amides than with the esters. Local anesthetics in the unprotonated form are poorly soluble in water and hence are often prepared as water-soluble salts, usually hydrochlorides. After injection, tissue buffers increase the pH of the solution, and some of the lipid-soluble base form of the drug is released [4].

Weak stereospecificity has been detected for some racemic pairs of local anesthetics, such as lidocaine derivatives [5].

III. PHARMACOKINETICS

The concentration of a local anesthetic in blood is determined by the amount of drug administered, the rate of absorption from the site of administration, the rate of tissue distribution, and the rate of metabolism and excretion [6]. Local anesthetics may modify their own disposition kinetics by dose-dependent effects on the cardiovascular system. For example, systemic exposure to these agents may alter hepatic blood flow and thereby alter clearance [7]. Patient factors such as age and disease state may also affect the pharmacokinetics of these drugs. Elimination half-lives may be prolonged two- to threefold in neonates [8]. Reduced clearance of lidocaine has been shown in patients with heart failure and in patients with cirrhosis of the liver.

In most situations these factors are not likely to be of major clinical importance as these drugs are administered directly at the site of action, although they may be of concern in cases of systemic toxicity [9].

A. Systemic Absorption

Local anesthetics are relatively lipid soluble compounds; therefore their diffusion across capillary membranes is not likely to be a rate-limiting step in their rate of absorption from the site of injection into the bloodstream. Absorption rates are thus related directly to local blood flow and inversely to local tissue binding [8].

Absorption of local anesthetics may be affected by a number of factors. The site of administration must be considered, with highly vascular areas favoring rapid absorption. Areas with large quantities of fat may sequester and delay the uptake of these drugs. The particular local anesthetic used is also important, because the various agents possess different local vasodilatory effects. For example, studies have shown that the intrinsic anesthetic potency of lidocaine is greater than that of mepivacaine, and in vitro the two drugs have a similar duration of action. However, in vivo, mepivacaine displays potency similar to that of lidocaine and has a longer duration of anesthesia. This is attributable to the greater vasodilator activity of lidocaine, resulting in greater absorption of this agent. For most of these drugs, a linear relationship exists between the dose of drug administered and the resultant peak blood concentration [10]. Slower speeds of injection result in lower peak blood levels.

A vasoconstrictor, such as epinephrine (adrenaline), may be added to reduce vascular absorption, thus prolonging the duration of anesthesia and decreasing the risk of systemic toxicity. The magnitude of this effect, however, will depend on the local anesthetic in question [3]. For example, the addition of epinephrine to lidocaine produces a much greater effect than that observed with the addition of epinephrine to prilocaine. This may be explained by the less pronounced intrinsic vasodilator action of prilocaine [11]. In general, the greatest effects of epinephrine are noted after intercostal blocks and with short-acting rather than long-acting agents [8].

B. Distribution

The distribution of local anesthetics can be characterized by a two- or three-compartment model [6]. In general, highly perfused organs such as the lung and kidney show higher concentrations of local anesthetics than less well perfused organs, indicating that the rate of tissue uptake is perfusion-limited [8,10]. Tissue uptake may also be affected by lipid solubility, with the more lipid-soluble drugs, such as etidocaine, being expected to have larger apparent volumes of distribution. The amount of unionized drug present (as determined by its pKa) will also be important, as it is this form that is most readily absorbed from the blood. Tissue protein binding may also play a significant role in determining tissue uptake [9]. The amide compounds are extensively protein-bound (55–95%), in particular to α_1-acid glycoprotein [1].

Due to their rapid breakdown, the tissue distribution of the ester group of local anesthetics has not been studied in any detail.

C. Metabolism

Local anesthetics of the ester type are hydrolysed by esterases, mainly in the blood (plasma pseudocholinesterase) but also in the liver, to paraminobenzoic acid (PABA) derivatives. These are excreted unchanged or as conjugated products in the urine [9]. The agents typically have very short plasma half-lives, for example, less than 1 minute for procaine and chloroprocaine. Degradation occurs with such rapidity that detection of these drugs in human blood after normal doses is difficult [7]. Inherent toxicity is thus less common for these agents [4], although the PABA derivatives appear to be responsible for hypersensitivity reactions, which occur in a small number of patients given anesthetics of this group [12]. A problem may occur when these agents are administered to individuals with atypical pseudocholinesterases.

In contrast, the amide-linked local anesthetics are primarily metabolized in the liver; N-dealkylation is followed by hydrolysis within the hepatic mixed function oxidase system [1,13]. Clearance of these drugs is limited by hepatic blood flow and hepatic function [9], although some breakdown of amide-type local anesthetics may occur in tissues other than the liver [10]. In general, more than 90% of these drugs are excreted as metabolites, primarily through the kidney, with a small proportion of parent drug appearing in the urine [14]. The half-lives of elimination (terminal phase) are typically measured in hours; for example, the half-life of lidocaine is 1.6 hours and that of bupivicaine is 3.5 hours [3].

IV. MECHANISM OF ACTION

Local anesthetics prevent the generation and conduction of nerve impulses. Their major mechanism of action involves interaction with specific binding sites within voltage-sensitive sodium channels. These binding sites are accessible only from the inner surface of nerve membrane; thus, the uncharged free base form of local anesthetics must initially traverse the nerve cell membrane [1]. Re-equilibration then takes place, generating more of the cationic form. The charged moiety is primarily responsible for neural blockade.

Local anesthetics decrease or prevent the large transient increase in permeability of excitable membranes to sodium produced by slight depolarization of the membrane [1]. Binding of the drug to its site of action prevents the sodium channel from opening by inhibiting the conformational changes that underlie channel activation. Physical blockade of the ion-conducting pore may play a role, but the contribution from this mechanism appears to be minor [6]. The effect of local anesthetics on potassium conduction is one-third to one-quarter of that on sodium conduction [13].

Local anesthetics cause reduction in the height and rate of rise of the action potential, as well as bringing about an elevation of the firing threshold and a slowing of the spread of conduction down the axon. The resting membrane potential, however, remains unchanged. With increasing concentrations of local anesthetic, total inhibition of conduction eventually occurs [13].

In mammals, two main types of fibers transmit pain impulses through peripheral nerves: A-d for acute sharp pain and C for chronic pain (see Chapter 2). Local anesthetics exert their action first on the A-d fibers.

A. Other Actions of Local Anesthetics

Most of these drugs exhibit a biphasic effect on vascular smooth muscle; that is, at extremely low concentrations vasoconstriction occurs, while at concentrations commonly used for regional anesthesia they tend to act as vasodilators [11]. Prilocaine provides the greatest enhancement of myogenic activity, whereas only minimal changes are seen with other anesthetics such as lidocaine [15,16]. The vascular effects may be related to competitive antagonism between local anesthetics and calcium ions in smooth muscle, following blockade of calcium ion entry channels by the cationic form of the drugs.

Antithrombotic effects of local anesthetics have been investigated in vivo [17,18]. One clinical study demonstrated the potential of lidocaine for the prevention of deep vein thrombosis [19].

Local anesthetics are able to suppress the adherence of leukocytes to the venular endothelium in vivo [20–23], which could suggest an anti-inflammatory action for these agents. In rabbits, for example, the dermal reaction provoked by irradiation (which involves a thrombotic and inflammatory response) was prevented or modified by local anesthetics [24].

V. STRUCTURE-ACTIVITY RELATIONSHIP

Certain physicochemical properties that are dependent on the chemical structure of the agents determine the activity of local anesthetics. The drugs may be characterized by their potency, latency of onset of action, and duration of action.

A. Potency

Intrinsic anesthetic potency, determined by in vitro techniques, is primarily dependent on lipid solubility. In vitro studies on isolated nerves show a correlation between the lipid (usually octanol):water partition coefficient of the agent and the minimum concentration necessary for conduction blockade. Highly lipid soluble compounds tend to penetrate the nerve membrane more easily, hence a lower extracellular concentration is required to block nerve conduction. For example, mepivacaine and prilocaine, which are poorly lipid soluble (partition coefficients of 0.8 and 0.9, respectively), are weaker anesthetic agents then etidocaine, which is substantially more lipophilic (partition coefficient 141) [11].

B. Onset of Action

Latency is determined by the rate of diffusion of the local anesthetic, which is correlated with the amount of drug present in the free base form. The pKa of the agent is thus an important factor affecting the speed of onset of anesthesia, as it is the uncharged species that penetrates through the membrane [10]. Drugs with a lower pKa (less basic) have a more rapid onset of action. The amides that have a rapid onset of action all have a pKa below 8 [3]. The lipophilicity and the concentration of the local anesthetic used may also affect the time to onset of anesthesia.

C. Duration of Action

The duration of action of local anesthetics is influenced by the degree of protein binding of the drug. More highly protein-bound local anesthetics would be expected to have a greater affinity for receptor sites and therefore to remain within the voltage-sensitive sodium channel for a longer period of time, leading to a longer duration of action. This observation is based on the relationship between the degree of plasma protein binding and the degree of binding to nerve membrane proteins [2,11]. Procaine, which is poorly bound to proteins (6%), demonstrates a relatively short duration of action (16 minutes) while bupivacaine, which is more highly protein bound (96%), displays a longer duration of action (125 minutes) [10,13]. Drugs with higher lipid solubility also tend to possess a longer duration of action, probably because of their partitioning into membrane structures [5].

Characteristics of local anesthetic action in vivo are not always well predicted by the structure and physicochemical properties of the compound determined in vitro. Numerous other factors, including interactions between the various properties as well as other pharmacological actions of the drugs, all affect clinical activity. For example, the duration of anesthesia may be altered by the intrinsic peripheral vascular effects of the local anesthetic.

D. Classification of Local Anesthetics

On the basis of differences in anesthetic potency and duration of action, local anesthetics can be divided into the following three groups [10]:

Group 1: Low potency and short duration of action (e.g. procaine)

Group 2: Intermediate potency and duration of action (e.g. lidocaine and prilocaine)

Group 3: High potency and long duration of action (e.g. bupivacaine)

VI. PHYSIOLOGICAL FACTORS INFLUENCING THE ACTION OF LOCAL ANESTHETICS

A. Effect of pH

As previously explained, pH determines the proportion of local anesthetic that is present as free base, according to the pKa of the particular agent. Under acidic conditions, the action of local anesthetics may be prolonged and potentiated. This is because the cationic form, which predominates at low pH, becomes trapped inside the nerve fibers, a phenomenon known as ion trapping [25].

B. Effect of Carbon Dioxide

Diffusion of carbon dioxide through the nerve membrane decreases the axoplasmic pH, thereby favoring the charged form of these drugs. Several attempts to enhance anesthetic action through the addition of carbon dioxide to local anesthetic solutions have been made. Carbon dioxide itself may depress neuronal excitability [6]. However, it is not certain whether this carbonation results in any advantage in terms of the onset of anesthesia under clinical conditions, although depth of block may be improved [11].

C. Effect of Vasoconstrictors

Vasoconstrictors, such as epinephrine, are commonly added to the local anesthetic preparations used in clinical practice. Their addition would be expected to lead to a local decrease in blood flow, thus reducing the rate of absorption into the circulation and retaining the local anesthetic at the desired site. These effects would eventually improve the depth and duration of anesthesia. Resultant blood concentrations are lower and thus systemic toxicity should also be less evident, allowing higher doses of the anesthetic to be used.

The effect of adding a vasoconstrictor is variable, depending on the particular local anesthetic involved. The increase in duration of action approaches 50% for short- and intermediate-acting agents, but is much less marked for long-acting compounds [26]. The site of administration also influences the ability of epinephrine to prolong anesthetic action.

VII. ADVERSE EFFECTS OF LOCAL ANESTHETICS

The safety margin of these drugs is low; however, their direct route of administration at the site of action and slow absorption from that site reduces systemic toxicity [13]. Systemic toxicity may occur as a result of the use of too high a dose or as a consequence of inadvertent intravascular injection of these agents. Other factors, such as the acid-base status, may also be of importance. Low pH or elevated pCO_2 levels may potentiate toxicity, as the amount of drug present in the more active ionized form is increased. The addition of a vasoconstrictor to the solution may lower potential toxicity by decreasing the rate of absorption of the local anesthetic from the site of administration.

A. Central Nervous System Toxicity

Local anesthetics readily cross the blood-brain barrier [25]. Central nervous system (CNS) toxicity is initially manifested by excitatory effects such as restlessness, tremors, and, ultimately, seizures. In general, the likelihood of convulsions being produced appears to be related directly to the local anesthetic potency of the particular agent [1]. At higher drug levels, local anesthetics may lead to CNS depression, resulting in respiratory arrest and death [13].

Local anesthetics act by depressing conduction in neuronal membranes as a result of sodium channel blockade. The biphasic effects on the CNS are attributed to an initial selective effect on the more sensitive inhibitory systems of the CNS, which results in CNS stimulation. This is followed by depression, caused by effects on the facilitatory systems [14].

B. Cardiovascular Toxicity

Cardiovascular effects of local anesthetics, manifested by hypotension, bradycardia, and cardiac arrhythmias, are usually seen only at high systemic concentrations, after effects on the CNS have taken place [1]. The drugs may exert their effect through a direct cardiac and peripheral vascular action as well as indirectly by conduction blockade of autonomic nerve fibers [25].

Depression of cardiac conduction may occur as a result of the interaction of local anesthetics with sodium channels. The maximal rate of increase of the cardiac action potential is depressed in a dose-dependent manner, resulting in slowed conduction of the action potential manifested by prolongation of the PR and QRS intervals. Re-entrant phenomena may develop with the sudden onset of ventricular arrhythmias [27]. Local anesthetics may also exert a dose-dependent inotropic action, depressing cardiac contractility to a degree proportional to their anesthetic potency [10]. Most local anesthetics cause a dose-dependent dilation of peripheral blood vessels [13]. The only agent that consistently induces vasoconstriction is cocaine [14].

C. Hypersensitivity Reactions

The incidence of allergic reactions to local anesthetics is low, accounting for approximately 1% of all untoward reactions to these drugs [28]. Hypersensitivity reactions are noted more commonly with local anesthetics of the ester type, such as procaine. Compounds of this group are metabolized to p-aminobenzoic acid derivatives that are thought to be responsible for these reactions. Manifestations are usually mild and include contact dermatitis, local swelling, rash, angioedema, asthma, fever, serum sickness syndrome, vasculitis, anaphylaxis, and circulatory collapse [29].

D. Methemoglobinemia

Large doses (greater than 10 mg/kg) of prilocaine may lead to the accumulation of the metabolite o-toluidine, an oxidizing agent capable of converting hemoglobin to methemoglobin. Clinically significant levels of methemoglobinemia may then result [6,12], particularly in infants. Methemoglobinemia is discussed in greater detail in Chapter 2.

E.   Local Tissue Toxicity

Local anesthetics rarely produced localized nerve damage at the concentrations used clinically [10]. Neurotoxic reactions following the use of large amounts of chloroprocaine have been attributed to the combination of low pH and sodium bisulfite that was added to the anesthetic solution [6]. Local neural damage may result from mechanical trauma following intraneural injection or contamination of the local anesthetic solution. Reversible skeletal muscle changes may follow intramuscular injection of these agents [25]. Tissue damage may be enhanced by the addition of epinephrine [30].

VIII.   PHARMACOLOGY OF THE LOCAL ANESTHETICS COMPRISING EMLA

A.   Lidocaine

Lidocaine (2-diethylaminoaceto-2′,6′-xylidide, Figure 2), an aminoethylamide, is a commonly used local anesthetic agent of the amino amide type. It is moderately lipid soluble with a pKa of 7.9 and plasma protein binding of about 64% [11,14]. Metabolism of lidocaine involves dealkylation in the liver by mixed function oxidases to monoethylglycine xylidide and glycine xylidide, which can then be metabolized further to monoethylglycine and xylidide. Monoethylglycine xylidide and glycine xylidide both retain some local anesthetic activity [1].

In terms of its local anesthetic properties, lidocaine demonstrates rapid onset and moderate duration of action [11]. It is more rapid in onset, twice as potent, and longer lasting than procaine, an amino ester drug [13]. Lidocaine exhibits a duration of action of approximately 1–2 hours for various regional anesthetic procedures [11]. The addition of epinephrine to lidocaine formulations decreases the rate of absorption and hence systemic toxicity, and prolongs the duration of action.

B.   Prilocaine

Prilocaine (2-propyl aminopropiono-*o*-toluidine, Figure 2) is also a member of the amino amide group of local anesthetics. Its pKa is identical to that of lidocaine, but it is not as lipid soluble and is only

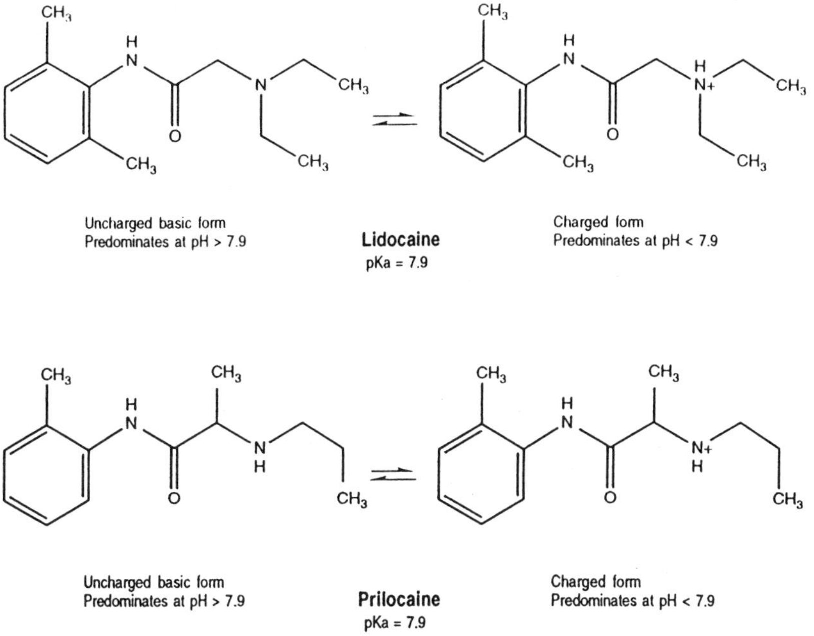

Figure 2 Free base and cationic forms of lidocaine and prilocaine.

approximately 55% bound to plasma proteins [14]. Prilocaine is metabolized in the liver, with the initial step of hydrolysis forming *o*-toluidine metabolites. The accumulation of these metabolites is believed to be responsible for the methemoglobinemia that has been noted after administration of large doses of this drug [1,12]. Prilocaine demonstrates the highest clearance of all the amide local anesthetics, and the possibility of a high degree of extrahepatic metabolism by the pulmonary and renal routes has been considered [8,9].

This local anesthetic provides a relatively rapid onset of action, moderate duration of anesthesia, and profound depth of conduction blockade [11]. In apparent contradiction to predicted structure–activity relationships, prilocaine, which is less lipid soluble and less protein bound than lidocaine, is of equal potency and has a longer duration of action. This inconsistency is best explained by the lack of vasodilatory activity of prilocaine compared to lidocaine, resulting in prilocaine being removed more slowly from the site of administration [7].

IX. CONCLUSION

The commonly used local anesthetics are chemical compounds with a basic structure consisting of an aromatic ring linked to an amine group. They may be divided into two groups, the amino esters and the amino amides. These drugs exert their local anesthetic effects through actions at sodium channels in the nerve membrane. Consideration of structure-activity relationships is important in assessing their efficacy, although other factors often need to be taken into account to explain in vivo observations.

REFERENCES

1. Ritchie JM, Greene NM: Local anesthetics. In: Goodman and Gilman's The Pharmacological Basis of Therapeutics. 8th edn. Goodman Gilman A, Goodman LS, Rall TW, Murad F, eds. Pergamon Press, New York. 1990: 311-331.
2. Hersch E, Condouris GA: Local anesthetics: a review of their pharmacology and clinical use. Compend Contin Educ Dent 1987; 8: 375-381.
3. Cousins MJ, Mather LE: Clinical pharmacology of local anaesthetics. Anaesth Intensive Care 1980; 8: 257-277.
4. Wildsmith JAW: Peripheral nerve and local anaesthetic drugs. Br J Anaesth 1986; 58: 692-700.
5. Courtney KR, Strichartz GR: Structural elements which determine local anesthetic activity. In: Handbook of Experimental Pharmacology: Local Anesthetics. Strichartz GR, ed. Springer-Verlag, Berlin. 1987: 165-186.
6. Strichartz GR, Covino BG: Local anesthetics. In: Anesthesia. 3rd edn. Miller RD, ed. Churchill-Livingstone, New York. 1990: 437-470.
7. Tucker GT, Mather LE: Clinical pharmacokinetics of local anaesthetics. Clin Pharmacokinetics 1979; 4: 241-278.
8. Tucker GT: Pharmacokinetics of local anaesthetics. Br J Anaesth 1986; 58: 717-731.

9. Arthur GR: Pharmacokinetics of local anesthetics. In: Handbook of Experimental Pharmacology: Local Anesthetics. Strichartz GR, ed. Springer-Verlag, Berlin. 1987: 165-186.

10. Covino BG: Pharmacology of local anesthetic agents. Rational Drug Ther 1987; 21: 1-9.

11. Covino BG: Pharmacology of local anaesthetic agents. Br J Anaesth 1986; 58: 701-716.

12. Hondeghem LM, Miller RD: Local anesthetics. In: Basic and Clinical Pharmacology. 4th edn. Katzung, ed. Appleton & Lange, East Norwalk, Conn. 1989: 315-322.

13. Carmichael FJ: Local anaesthetics. In: Principles of Medical Pharmacology. 5th edn. Kalant H, Roschlau WHE, eds. BC Decker, Toronto. 1989: 237-243.

14. Stanton-Hicks MD: Local anesthetics: pharmacology and clinical applications. Hosp Formul 1987; 22: 156-171.

15. Sanders HD: The vasoconstrictor and vasodilator effects of procaine. Can J Physiol Pharmacol 1965; 43: 39.

16. Blair MR: Cardiovascular pharmacology of local anaesthetics. Br J Anaesth 1975; 47: 247-252.

17. Luostarinen V, Evers H, Lyytikäinen M-T, Scheinin A, Wahlen A: Antithrombotic effects of lidocaine and related compounds on laser-induced microvascular injury. Acta Anaesth Scand 1981; 25: 9-11.

18. Blair WF, Greene ER, Edridge M, Cipoletti R: Hemodynamics after microsurgical anastomosis. J Microsurg 1981; 2: 157-164.

19. Cooke ED, Bowcock SA, Lloyd MJ, Pilcher MF: Intravenous lignocaine in prevention of deep vein thrombosis after elective hip surgery. Lancet 1977; 797-799.

20. Giddon DB, Lindhe J: In vivo quantitation of local anesthetic suppression of leukocyte adherence. Am J Pathol 1972; 68: 327-338.

21. MacGregor RR, Thorner RE, Wright DM: Lidocaine inhibits granulocyte adherence and prevents granulocyte delivery to inflammatory sites. Blood 1980; 56: 203-209.

22. Paul H, Clayburne G, Schumacher HR: Lidocaine inhibits leucocyte migration and phagocytosis in monosodium urate crystal-induced synovitis in dogs. J Rheumatol 1983; 10: 434-439.

23. Behnia R, Wilkinson CJ: Lidocaine treatment of experimental cutaneous lesions from potassium chloride injection. Anaesthesiology 1977; 47: 428-429.

24. Ohlsen L, Evers H, Segerstrom K, Hagelqist A, Graffman S: Local anaesthetics modifying the dermal response of irradiation. Acta Oncol 1987; 26: 467-476.
25. Conception M, Covino BG: Rational use of local anaesthetics. Drugs 1984; 27: 256-270.
26. Murphy MF: Local anesthetic agents. Emerg Med Clin North Am 1988; 6: 769-776.
27. Reiz S, Nath S: Cardiotoxicity of local anaesthetic agents. Br J Anaesth 1986; 58: 736-746.
28. Bennet CR: Anesthetic complication and office emergencies. In: Monheim's Local Anesthesia and Pain Control in Dental Practice. 7th edn. CV Mosby, St Louis. 1984: 225.
29. McCaughey W: Adverse effects of local anaesthetics. Drug Safety 1992; 7: 178-189.
30. Selander D: Ph.D. thesis.

2

Clinical Pharmacology and Toxicology of EMLA

Pascale Burtin

Robert Debré Children's Hospital
Paris, France

Shinya Ito

The Hospital for Sick Children
Toronto, Ontario, Canada

I. INTRODUCTION

The clinical need for a topically applied local anesthetic suitable for use on intact skin has been recognized for many years. Investigations into the efficacy of topically applied local anesthetics were first carried out in 1957 [1]. These and later investigations [2,3] demonstrated that the preparations of local anesthetics available at that time did not penetrate skin sufficiently to provide clinically effective anesthesia.

Since then, many formulations have been tested. Dimethyl sulfoxide, dimethyl acetamide, and other aprotic solvents were used to increase permeation of local anesthetics into the skin [4]. Although these formulations could induce anesthesia, their clinical use was limited because of severe local reactions to the solvents [5,6]. In addition, the efficacy of the anesthetic was reduced owing to the strong affinity of these agents for the solvent. A formulation of 10% ketocaine (a highly lipophilic amino-ether local anesthetic) in a vehicle comprising isopropanol, glycerol, and water was extensively investigated and provided effective analgesia [7,8], but its use was also discontinued following local reactions, which included blistering [8]. A 30% lidocaine patch was similarly discontinued, as the high concentration of the drug increased toxicity [9].

The skin is composed of two main layers: the epidermis and the dermis. The epidermis is made up of squamous epithelial keratinocytes, which form a surface protective barrier called the stratum corneum, the thickness of which varies throughout the body. The epidermis is devoid of blood vessels and nerves, and has little or no sensory function. The dermis, on the other hand, is rich in blood vessels, and has a variety of sensory nerves and nerve endings. Light touch is transmitted by fast-conducting A-b fibers, cold and pinprick by fast A-d fibers. Warmth, dull pain, and unpleasant mechanical or thermal stimuli are conducted by slower, unmyelinated C fibers [10].

Topically applied local anesthetic agents must be able to penetrate through the epidermis to act on sensory nerve endings in the dermis in order to provide effective anesthesia. Formulations must provide a high water content (which softens the stratum corneum, making it more penetrable) together with a high proportion of the lipophilic, unionized (basic) form of the anesthetic, which is membrane permeable. If the basic form of an anesthetic, such as lidocaine, is dissolved in oil and an oil-in-water (10:90) emulsion prepared, this provides a high water content and a high proportion of the basic form. However, the maximum concentration of lidocaine that is possible to dissolve in the oil droplets is about 20%, giving an overall concentration of 2%, which is not sufficient to induce analgesia—particularly as the anesthetic is not easily released from association with the oil.

II. EMLA

EMLA® (eutectic mixture of local anesthetics) cream essentially provides all the requirements for skin penetration, with none of the drawbacks. It is composed of an oil-in-water emulsion of lidocaine and prilocaine local anesthetics. Rather than relying on an oil solvent to dissolve the anesthetics, EMLA cream utilizes the eutectic mixture of the two compounds. Solids can interact to form a uniform mixture that has a lower melting point than the components, without any chemical change to the components. A eutectic mixture occurs at the ratio of solids that provides the lowest possible melting point. Pure lidocaine and pure prilocaine have melting points above room temperature (67 and 37°C, respectively), but a 1:1 ratio mixture of the two has a melting point of about 18°C, and is thus normally liquid at room temperature. EMLA cream is prepared by emulsifying this oily liquid in water to give a final concentration of 25 mg/g lidocaine and 25 mg/g prilocaine. The cream is stabilized by a polyoxyethylene castor oil emulsifier (Arlatone®), thickened with Carbopol® and the pH adjusted to about 9. Although the final proportion of anesthetic in the cream is only 5%, which reduces the possibility of toxicity, the oil droplets within the emulsion are composed of 80% anesthetic, which provides a highly effective analgesic concentration [10-12]. In addition, the high water content of the cream provides good hydration of the skin, which aids absorption.

EMLA cream was developed for use primarily on intact skin, but it has also been found to produce effective topical analgesia of lacerated skin and mucous membranes prior to a variety of clinical procedures. The usual recommendation is to apply 1–2.5 g of the cream per 10 cm^2 of skin under an occlusive dressing for various periods of time. Ineffective occlusion may cause evaporation of water, resulting in incomplete hydration of the stratum corneum and thus decreased absorption of the eutectic mixture. In addition to the cream, EMLA is available as a patch (see Chapter 5) and a sterile cream (see Chapter 11).

III. PHARMACODYNAMICS

A. Dose-Response

A dose-response study in healthy volunteers showed that the concentration of the eutectic lidocaine/prilocaine oil in the emulsified cream must be at least 5% [11]. At this concentration, the magnitude of dermal analgesia was relatively constant among individuals after applications of at least 1 g of cream per 10 cm^2 skin for 1 hour [11]. The efficacy of a "thick" layer (2.0 $g/10$ cm^2) of EMLA cream was compared to that of a "thin" layer (0.5 $g/10$ cm^2) in a randomized study involving 100 children undergoing venipuncture [13]. No child in either group experienced moderate or severe pain, but more children in the study group treated with the thinner layer were assessed as experiencing slight pain. In a study conducted in patients undergoing the cutting of split-skin grafts, a dose of 1.5 g EMLA cream per 10 cm^2 appeared to be sufficient to provide analgesia, when application times varied between 2 and 5 hours [14].

B. Duration of Application

The duration of application of EMLA cream is very important. The main factor on which the application time depends is the structure of the skin to which it is applied, because the local anesthetics must first penetrate through the epidermis, then diffuse down to the dermis and permeate the nerve cell membranes before exerting any analgesic effect. In intact skin, the duration of application required can vary according to the local blood flow and the thickness of the layers of skin, but it is generally at least 60 minutes. Shorter application times are required in areas of skin lesions, where the epidermis is not an effective barrier, or on mucous membranes, which do not possess a keratinized layer of cells.

Intact Skin

The influence of application time on dermal analgesia has been studied in a number of double-blind, randomized trials. Early studies showed that, in healthy volunteers, an application time of at least 60 minutes under an occlusive dressing was desirable, and an increased effect plus even more reliable dermal analgesia were achieved with application times of 90 or 120 minutes. In most instances, the duration of effective analgesia was more than 2 hours after removal of the cream [11,12].

Arendt-Nielsen and Bjerring [15] used laser-induced pain to evaluate the analgesia provided by the application of 2 g/10 cm^2 of EMLA cream for different periods of time (15 to 120 minutes) on the dorsum of the hand. When EMLA cream was applied for 15 minutes, both sensory and pain thresholds increased, but total pain blockade was not achieved. The analgesic effect of EMLA cream increased with longer application times (see Table 1); after a 2-hour application the effect was similar to that produced by conventional lidocaine 1% infiltration.

With application times less than or equal to 60 minutes, the analgesic effect of EMLA cream continued to increase after removal of the cream [15]; continuation of effect was also observed by Evers et al. [11]. These observations suggest that the epidermis may act as a reservoir for local anesthetics. After the cream is removed, the local anesthetics continue to diffuse from the epidermis into deeper layers

Table 1 Pain and Sensory Blockade After Application of 2 g/cm^2 of EMLA on the Dorsum of the Hand, According to Arendt-Nielsen et al. [15]

Length of application (minutes)	Time of onset of pain blockade after removal of the cream (minutes)	Duration of the pain blockade (minutes)	Total sensory blockade reached
15	–	0	No
30	30	60	No
60	15	75	No
80	0	100	Yes
100–120	0	120–140	Yes

of the skin and reach the nerve endings. This phenomenon is important because it may be of practical interest, allowing a wide margin of analgesic efficacy during which procedures can be carried out after removal of the cream. This may be particularly useful in outpatient clinics.

Clinical studies of pain relief for venipuncture in both adults and children showed that EMLA analgesia reaches optimal levels after 45 to 60 minutes of application [16,17]. However, some patients showed a significant relief of pain, in comparison with placebo, with application times as short as 5 minutes [16,18]. In children, two double-blind, placebo-controlled studies [19,20] found no difference in analgesia between short (20 and 30 minutes, respectively) and long (75 and 300 minutes) application times. An application time of less than 60 minutes was also found to be satisfactory for the curettage of molluscum contagiosum in children [21].

For cutting split skin grafts, application times of at least 1 to 1.5 hours are necessary to obtain adequate analgesia; however, the anesthetic effect decreases for application times longer than 3 hours. This may be explained by a depletion of the anesthetic oil droplets in the layer of EMLA cream closest to the skin surface, and suggests that the bandage should be massaged to homogenize the cream during longer applications ([22]; see Chapter 15).

A study by Cesany and Raska [23] used an electromyograph (EMG) device to measure the superficial skin sensibility threshold and speed of sensory fibers with EMLA cream or mesocaine gel anesthesia. For both agents, maximal effect was obtained within 45 to 60 minutes after application. The sensibility threshold decreased after 20 to 30 minutes, then later increased by an average of 1 milliamp. The anesthetics unexpectedly reduced the conduction speed of sensory fibers by 2 to 4 milliseconds.

There are local differences in the onset and duration of action of EMLA cream; variations occur according to the area of body to which it is applied. The onset of action of EMLA is mainly influenced by local epidermal and dermal thickness. The duration of action depends on the rate of diffusion of the anesthetics into the surrounding tissues and the systemic circulation, and is thus influenced by local blood flow [24-26].

Absorption of the local anesthetics is more rapid and more extensive from the skin of the face than from that of the forearm. However, the analgesic efficacy on facial skin appears to vary considerably between individuals, with some subjects experiencing no or only slight analgesic effect. Differences in local blood flow probably contribute to this variability. Application for 30 minutes is sufficient to provide analgesia in those patients who are susceptible to the cream; efficacy decreases with longer application times [25]. In the cubital fossa and on the hand, onset of analgesia is delayed, although efficacy continues to increase for 60 minutes after cream removal and declines only slowly. This pattern is probably due to the thick epidermis and poor blood flow. On the back, onset is rapid but analgesia wanes immediately after removal of the cream. The thick dermis at this location might be able to absorb and redistribute a larger volume of the anesthetics, so that the amount or concentration of EMLA cream applied to the back may be insufficient [26].

One study in a limited number of subjects suggested a clinically significant difference in both the onset of action and the density of pain block in black- versus white-skinned patients [35]. Following identical application times of EMLA cream, pain relief was 20 to 30% less in black patients, which may be explained by an increased density of the stratum corneum and by sequestration of local anesthetics in the melanosomes. Additional studies are needed to elucidate whether longer application times would increase the efficacy of EMLA cream in black patients.

Diseased Skin

In the atopic skin and on psoriatic plaques, an application time of 15 minutes appears sufficient to produce analgesia, but the effect persists for only 15 to 30 minutes. This rapid but shorter analgesia is probably explained by an enhanced penetration of the anesthetics into the dermis and hypodermis, and a higher cutaneous blood flow resulting in a faster vascular uptake of the analgesics [28]. On the other hand, longer application times (about 60 minutes) were found to be necessary for cleansing leg ulcers [29], probably because of the aggressive nature of the procedure.

Mucous Membranes

In contrast to the skin, mucous membranes offer less protection of nerve endings and allow faster penetration of local anesthetics, resulting in faster onset of action. However, higher vascular flow allows faster clearance, resulting in a more rapid decline of analgesia.

Analgesic properties of EMLA cream on the oral mucosa vary according to the site of application. The sensory and pain threshold on labial gingiva was assessed in healthy volunteers using electrical stimulation [30]. After application of EMLA cream for 4 minutes, maximal analgesic effect was observed after 5–20 minutes and the pain returned to control levels 30 minutes after removal of the cream. Thus, it would be possible to perform only small and relatively short surgical procedures using EMLA analgesia. The intensity and duration of analgesia in this study [30] were similar to those produced by 10% lidocaine spray. In another study [31], which used laser stimulation, application of EMLA cream (1 g) for 2 minutes on the gingiva produced adequate analgesia for 10 minutes; the maximal pain threshold was reached immediately after removal of the cream.

EMLA cream could be useful in providing analgesia for needle insertion in some areas of the mouth. An application time of 2 minutes was found to be sufficient to produce a high degree of analgesia to a depth of 2 mm in the lower buccal fold [32] and to a depth of 5 mm in the buccal sulcus of the upper premolar region [33]. When pain thresholds were tested using laser stimulation on the tongue, an application time of 5 minutes was sufficient to produce adequate analgesia; prolongation of the application time to 15 minutes improved the analgesic efficacy and duration [31]. However, in the palatal area, pain could not be totally blocked for needle insertion with application times of up to 5 minutes [32].

The time of onset of EMLA-induced analgesia of the vulval mucosa is 5–7 minutes. An application time of 10 minutes produced satisfactory anesthesia for the cautery of condylomata acuminata in 92% of patients ($n = 12$), but longer application times (15 to 20 minutes) resulted in decreased efficacy [34]. In men, application times of 20–70 minutes allowed pain-free cautery of genital warts [35]. Chapter 10 discusses the use of EMLA cream for these indications in greater detail.

C.   Depth of Analgesia

The depth of analgesia to needle insertion in the forearm was determined in healthy volunteers [24]. The sensory and pain threshold depths increased linearly with increasing application times of EMLA cream (30, 60, 90, and 120 minutes). Analgesia progressed further into deeper layers of the skin after removal of the cream. The maximal depth of analgesia was 5 mm, which exceeds the mean skin thickness. This was observed 30 minutes after a 90-minute application, and for a 60-minute period following a 120-minute application.

D.   Miscellaneous Properties of EMLA

Skin application of EMLA cream before blood sampling does not distort the results of common clinical chemistry and hematology measurements [36].

EMLA cream has been shown to inhibit adrenaline-induced sweating in healthy volunteers following an application time of 1 hour [37]. It is effective in reducing pruritus induced by histamine and artificial pruritogenes, probably because the itching sensation is mediated by the neural pathways that are responsible for pain [38]. A preliminary study to investigate the efficacy of EMLA cream in treating post-herpatic neuralgia showed that pain was reduced 6 to 10 hours after removal of the cream, following a 24-hour application period [39]. In rabbits, EMLA cream has been shown to inhibit the inflammatory reaction of the skin after irradiation [40].

IV.   SYSTEMIC ABSORPTION

The rationale of topical anesthesia is to obtain a high concentration of the active components at the target site, while keeping systemic exposure as low as possible. Systemic exposure is directly correlated with the dose and the systemic bioavailability and is inversely correlated with clearance rate (see Chapter 1).

Prilocaine and lidocaine have been used for many years, and adverse event profiles for the individual agents are well established. Prilocaine can induce methemoglobinemia, via its *o*-toluidine metabolite. Lidocaine, which can be used therapeutically for the treatment of cardiac dysrhythmia at plasma levels ranging from 1 to 6 µg/ml, can induce ventricular fibrillation or cardiac arrest on overdose [41]. In addition, concentrations of both lidocaine and prilocaine above 6 µg/ml may be associated with symptoms of central nervous system toxicity such as sleepiness, dizziness, paresthesias, and seizures.

Drug absorption from the skin is variable, depending on the location and the state of the skin barrier. The absorption of lidocaine and prilocaine after dermal application of EMLA cream to normal skin is low, and generally plasma concentrations of these anesthetics do not even approach levels that are known to exert pharmacological or toxicological effects. Blood concentrations of the two components have similar profiles, but prilocaine concentrations are consistently lower than those of lidocaine [42].

A. Plasma Concentrations of Lidocaine and Prilocaine

Intact Skin

The application of EMLA cream (20 g) for 1 hour to adult volunteers resulted in maximum plasma concentrations of lidocaine and prilocaine of 0.180 µg/ml and 0.067 µg/ml, respectively, 2 to 3 hours after application [11]. These are well below the plasma concentrations known to induce toxic effects, i.e. approximately 6 µg/ml for both lidocaine and prilocaine. In another study, application of EMLA cream (10 g over a 100 cm^2 area) on the forearm or the face for 2 hours gave a negligible plasma lidocaine concentration, and prilocaine was undetectable [42].

Even after prolonged application times over large areas, such as during use of EMLA cream for cutting split skin grafts, blood concentrations of lidocaine and prilocaine remain low. Ohlsén et al. [22] used application times of 1.5 to 7.6 hours over areas from 50 to over 1000 cm^2. The maximum individual concentration of lidocaine (1.1 µg/ml) and prilocaine (0.2 µg/ml) were recorded with an application area of 1296 cm^2. In this study, reported in more detail in Chapter 15, the blood concentrations of lidocaine and prilocaine increased with the size and duration of application for up to 5 hours, after which the levels decreased even in the presence of the cream on the skin.

Diseased Skin

After application of 4 to 6 g of EMLA cream on diseased skin of patients with psoriasis or atopic dermatitis, the plasma concentrations of both anesthetics increased more rapidly and reached higher levels than were found for normal skin, while remaining 100 times lower than those associated with toxicity [42]. Application of 10 g of 2% EMLA cream (an experimental concentration not commercially available) for 60 minutes to leg ulcers resulted in negligible blood levels of lidocaine and prilocaine. It was found that approximately 15% of the dose of prilocaine reached the systemic circulation [29]. Application of 10 g of 5% EMLA sterile cream on leg ulcers resulted in maximal plasma concentrations of 0.84 µg/ml for lidocaine and 0.08 µg/ml for prilocaine [43].

Mucous Membranes

The systemic absorption of lidocaine and prilocaine from EMLA cream applied to gingival mucosa was investigated in healthy volunteers [30] and in patients undergoing removal of arch bars [44]. Plasma concentrations were measured at 5, 10, 20, and 30 minutes after application of 4 g of EMLA cream for 4 minutes. The highest individual plasma concentration was 0.47 µg/ml at 5 minutes for lidocaine and 0.21 µg/ml at 10 minutes for prilocaine. Absorption of the local anesthetics was more rapid than after application of a 10% lidocaine spray, while there was no difference between the two methods in producing analgesia [30]. In patients receiving supplementary infiltration of 36 mg lidocaine, plasma concentrations remained below 1 µg/ml [44].

Children

Various agents have been found to have a higher permeability through infants' skin in comparison with that of older children and adults. However, very low levels of local anesthetics have been measured in infants after application of EMLA cream. Nilsson [45] and Engberg [46] found low plasma concentrations of local anesthetics in 22 infants aged 3 to 12 months and 10 infants younger than 3 months of age, after application of a standard dose of 2 g of EMLA cream on a skin area of 16 cm^2 (maximum plasma concentrations: lidocaine 0.41 µg/ml, prilocaine 0.13 µg/ml). These levels were similar to those found in adults given a dosage 10 times greater, over an application area 20 times greater.

Similarly, in children over 2 years of age, systemic exposure to the anesthetics was low after application of doses up to 16 g (or 0.8 g/kg) of EMLA cream [47,48]. Bruguerolle et al. measured levels of lidocaine in infants aged 32 months after application of 0.5 g/kg EMLA cream to the cubital fossae for 1 hour [49]. Following application in the morning, plasma levels were found to be significantly higher than those measured after an evening application. These circadian variations may be partly explained by an increased cutaneous temperature in the afternoon corresponding to the well-known circadian rhythm of body temperature.

V.   SYSTEMIC TOXICITY

Toxic levels of lidocaine and prilocaine do not appear to have been reached in any of the reported studies of EMLA cream, although application to large areas or on diseased skin gives rise to higher levels than seen under other conditions of use. Therefore, systemic toxicity related to high blood levels is not likely to occur, except under exceptional circumstances. The only systemic complication that has been reported to date is methemoglobinemia in infants.

A.   Methemoglobinemia

Two of the metabolites of prilocaine, 4-hydroxy-2-methyl aniline and *o*-toluidine, are capable of oxidizing hemoglobin to methemoglobin; thus, EMLA cream has the potential risk of inducing methemoglobinemia.

Normal methemoglobin levels, expressed as a percentage of total hemoglobin, range between 0.08 and 4.7% in premature newborns, 0 and 2.8% in term newborns, and 0 and 2.4% in infants and children [50]. Normally, the small amount of naturally formed methemoglobin is reduced to hemoglobin in healthy adults and children. The rate-limiting step in this process is the enzyme NADH-methemoglobin reductase. The amount of this enzyme in umbilical cord blood is only 40 to 60% of adult values; levels increase to those of adults within the first 3 months of life. Infants are thus at increased risk of developing methemoglobinemia when exposed to oxidizing agents.

The increased potential risk of methemoglobinemia has led to EMLA cream's being contraindicated in infants under 3 months old. However, there is certainly a need for topical anesthetics during the neonatal period, and more studies should be conducted to quantify the exact rate and extent of this potential problem.

To date, only one clinically significant case of methemoglobinemia (methemoglobin concentration of 28%) has been reported following use of EMLA cream [51]. This occurred with a prilocaine dose of 23.6 mg/kg applied for 5 hours in a 12-week-old premature infant who received concomitant trimethoprim-sulphamethoxazole, a therapy that is also capable of inducing methemoglobin formation. This case has been widely and erroneously publicized as proof of the danger of EMLA cream to the newborn, even when applied in recommended doses.

Subsequently, three prospective studies designed to investigate methemoglobin levels have been conducted in children and infants [45,46,52]. In 22 infants aged 3 to 12 months, 2 g of EMLA cream was applied to a 16 cm^2 area of skin for a period of 4 hours. Methemoglobin levels, assessed up to 8 hours after the application, were all within a normal range (the maximum individual value was 2%). However, there was a significant increase in methemoglobin in infants aged between 3 and 6 months, when compared to the individual baseline values [46].

In another study, infants younger than 3 months received 2 g of EMLA cream [45]. Results showed a statistically significant but clinically unimportant increase in plasma methemoglobin levels (the maximum individual value was 3.4%). As expected, methemoglobin reductase activity in erythrocytes did not reach adult levels until after the age of 3 months. The activity of this enzyme was inversely correlated with maximum methemoglobin values, but there was no correlation between methemoglobin levels and the very low concentrations of prilocaine detected in the blood.

Methemoglobin levels were also assessed over a 24-hour period in 48 healthy children aged 1 to 6 years, after a 2-hour application of

EMLA cream (5 g) [52]. The peak methemoglobin levels remained well within safe limits (< 1%), although the concentrations were significantly higher than those of a control group. Frayling et al. emphasized that methemoglobin levels remained slightly elevated 24 hours after administration of EMLA cream, suggesting that cumulative effects may occur in children receiving the cream on a daily basis.

Studies conducted to date suggest that EMLA cream can be used safely in infants over 3 months, provided certain precautions are observed, i.e. that no concomitant therapy with another methemoglobin-inducing agent (such as sulfa drugs) is given, the total amount of cream applied is 2 g or less, and applications are not repeated too frequently. More data on the safety profile of EMLA cream in newborns and infants younger than 3 months are needed. Until further clinical data are available, EMLA cream should be used with caution in such patients.

B. Inner Ear Toxicity

Inner ear damage is a potential risk with all forms of local anesthetics approaching the middle ear. Studies in laboratory animals have shown that instillation of EMLA cream into the round window niche caused functional impairment and morphological damage to the organ of Corti in the basal coil [53]. Instillation into the external auditory canal with an intact tympanic membrane caused no morphological changes in either the middle or the inner ear, and there was no audiometric evidence of ototoxicity in 29 patients undergoing tympanic membrane anesthesia for myringotomy and ventilation tube insertion [54].

Little data regarding the ototoxic potential of EMLA cream in humans are available. However, when applied on the intact tympanic membrane, EMLA cream is probably at least as safe as the usual forms of local anesthetics [55] (see Chapter 14).

VI. LOCAL REACTIONS

A. Blanching and Erythema

When applied on the skin for 0.5 to 2 hours, EMLA cream gives rise to blanching (pallor) with no local irritation [24]. This initial response may be followed by erythema (redness) 1 to 2 hours after removal of the cream. On prolonged exposure (more than 2 to 3 hours) the skin becomes erythematous at the end of the application period [24]. Placebo cream causes blanching but no subsequent erythema. The time-dependent biphasic effects of EMLA cream may be due to concentration-dependent effects of the anesthetics on vascular smooth muscle. At very low concentrations (e.g. short application times), they may produce vascular contraction, while at higher concentrations, which would occur after long application times, the anesthetics relax vascular and bronchial smooth muscle and could thus induce erythema [56].

In patients with atopic and eczematous skin lesions, EMLA cream results in blanching after 5 to 15 minutes of application, and an erythematous lesion sometimes surrounded by a 2- to 3-mm white border after application for 0.5 to 1.0 hours. Localized purpura was also reported in one eczematous patient [27]. Coupled with the fact that patients with various skin lesions achieve abnormally high serum concentrations of lidocaine and prilocaine after topical application, the abnormal skin reactions to EMLA cream in these patients may be due partly to enhanced penetration of the anesthetics into the dermis/hypodermis resulting in higher tissue concentrations of the anesthetics.

As a result of these local vascular reactions, EMLA cream can affect intradermal skin test results, thus precluding it from use in these tests [57], although the weal response and delayed-type hypersensitivity reactions are reportedly unaffected [58,59].

B. Repeated Applications of EMLA Cream and Local Reactions

EMLA cream was used in 31 hemodialysis patients for alleviation of cannulation pain for a period of 1 to 1.5 years [60]. Each patient received 300 to 312 applications of the cream during this period. There was no correlation between the number of applications and local reactions, which were mild in most cases. Only two patients discontinued EMLA treatment because of local irritation—one with severe psoriasis and one because of irritation due to the Tegaderm® dressing. No tolerance to the analgesic effect developed, even after 150 applications of EMLA cream to the same skin areas.

VII. CONCLUSION

EMLA, containing 5% lidocaine and prilocaine in a cream, has been shown to produce effective topical analgesia of the skin and the mucous membranes for a wide spectrum of superficial procedures. Recommendations are to apply EMLA cream under occlusion for 60 to 120 minutes on intact skin, and for a few to 30 minutes on mucous membranes and diseased skin. Duration of analgesia is about 2 hours on intact skin and 30 minutes on mucous membranes. Systemic absorption of lidocaine and prilocaine from the cream is extremely low, resulting in a wide safety margin. However, caution should be taken with large applications or on diseased skin, and, because of methemoglobin formation induced by metabolites of prilocaine, in infants less than 3 months old.

REFERENCES

1. Monash S: Topical anaesthesia of the unbroken skin. Arch Dermatol 1957; 76: 752-756.
2. Adriani G, Dalili H: Penetration of local anesthetics through epithelial barriers. Anesth Analg (Cleve) 1971; 50: 834.
3. Dalili H, Adriani G: The efficacy of local anaesthetics in blocking the sensations of itch, burning and pain in normal and "sunburned" skin. Clin Pharmacol Ther 1971; 12: 913.
4. Brechner VL, Cohen DD, Pretsky I: Dermal anesthesia by the topical application of tetracaine base dissolved in dimethyl sulphoxide. Ann NY Acad Sci 1967; 141: 524-531.
5. Kligman AM: Topical pharmacology and toxicology of dimethyl sulphoxide. J Am Med Assoc 1965; 193: 140.
6. Rubin LF: Toxicity of dimethyl sulphoxide, alone and in combination. Ann NY Acad Sci 1975; 243: 98-103.
7. Âkerman B: Percutaneous local anaesthesia. Problems—solutions. Acta Anaesthesiol Scand 1978; 70 (suppl): 90-91.
8. Pontén B, Ohlsén L: Skin surface application of ketocaine to provide local anaesthesia for cutting split skin grafts. Br J Plast Surg 1977; 30: 251-254.

9. Lubens HM, Ausdenmoore RW, Shafer AD, Reece RM: Anesthetic patch for painful procedures such as minor operations. Am J Dis Child 1974; 128: 192-194.

10. Freeman JA, Doyle E, Tee NG, Morton NS: Topical anaesthesia of the skin: a review. Paediatr Anaesth 1993; 3: 129-138.

11. Evers H, Von Dardel O, Juhlin L, Ohlsen L, Vinnars E: Dermal effects of compositions based on the eutectic mixture of lignocaine and prilocaine. Br J Anaesth 1985; 57: 997-1005.

12. Juhlin L, Evers H: EMLA: a new topical anesthetic. Adv Dermatol 1990; 5: 75-92.

13. Sims C: Thickly and thinly applied lignocaine-prilocaine cream prior to venipuncture in children. Anaesth Intens Care 1991; 19: 343-345.

14. Lähteenmäki T, Lillieborg S, Ohlsén L, Olenius M, Strömbeck JO: Topical analgesia for the cutting of split-skin grafts: a multicenter comparison of two doses of a lidocaine/prilocaine cream. Plast Reconstr Surg 1988; 82: 458-462.

15. Arendt-Nielsen L, Bjerring P: Laser-induced pain for evaluation of local analgesia: a comparison of topical application (EMLA) and local injection (lidocaine). Anesth Analg 1988; 67: 115-123.

16. Ehrenström-Reiz G, Reiz S, Stockman O: Topical anesthesia with EMLA, a new lidocaine prilocaine cream and the cusum technique for detection of minimal application time. Acta Anaesthesiol Scand 1983; 27: 510-512.

17. Hallen B, Olsson JL, Uppfeldt A: Pain-free venipuncture. Effect of timing of application of local anesthetic cream. Anaesthesia 1984; 39: 969-972.

18. Nott MR, Peacock JL: Relief of injection pain in adults. EMLA cream for 5 minutes before venipuncture. Anaesthesia 1990; 45: 772-774.

19. Dolwitz A, Uppfeldt A: Schmerzlinderung bei Venenpunktion: Applikationszeit und Wirksamkeit einer Lidocain-Prilocain-Creme. Anaesthesist 1985; 34: 355-358.

20. Hopkins CS, Buckley CJ, Bush GH: Pain-free injection in infants: use of a lignocaine-prilocaine cream to prevent pain at intravenous induction of general anesthesia in 1 to 5-year-old children. Anaesthesia 1988; 43: 198-201.

21. de Waard-van der Spek FB, Oranje AP, Lillieborg S, Wim CJ, Stolz E: Treatment of molluscum contagiosum using a lidocaine/prilocaine cream (EMLA) for analgesia. J Am Acad Dermatol 1990; 23: 685-688.

22. Ohlsén L, Englesson S, Evers H: An anaesthetic lidocaine/prilocaine cream (EMLA) for epicutaneous application tested for cutting split skin grafts. Scand J Plast Reconstr Surg 1985; 19: 201-219.

23. Cesany P, Raska D: Skin graft harvesting under local anaesthesia. Acta Chir Plast 1990; 32: 11-15.

24. Bjerring P, Arendt-Nielsen L: Depth and duration of skin analgesia to needle insertion after topical application of EMLA cream. Br J Anaesth 1990; 64: 173-177.

25. Nielsen JC, Arendt-Nielsen L, Bjerring P, Svensson P: The analgesic effect of EMLA on facial skin. Acta Derm Venereol 1992; 72: 281-284.

26. Arendt-Nielsen L, Bjerring P, Nielsen J: Regional variations in analgesic efficacy of EMLA cream quantitatively evaluated by argon laser stimulation. Acta Derm Venereol 1990; 70: 314-318.

27. Hymes JA, Spraker MK: Racial differences in the effectiveness of a topically applied mixture of local anesthetics. Regional Anesth 1986; 11: 11-13.

28. Juhlin L, Rollman O: Vascular effects of a local anesthetic mixture in atopic dermatitis. Acta Derm Venereol 1984; 64: 439-440.

29. Enander Malmros I, Nilsen T, Lillieborg S: Plasma concentrations and analgesic effect of EMLA (lidocaine/prilocaine) cream for the cleansing of leg ulcers. Acta Derm Venereol 1990; 70: 227-230.

30. Haasio J, Jokinen T, Numminen M, Rosenberg PH: Topical anaesthesia of gingival mucosa by 5% eutectic mixture of lignocaine and prilocaine or by 10% lignocaine spray. Br J Oral Maxillofacial Surg 1990; 28: 99-101.

31. Svensson P, Bjerring P, Arendt-Nielsen L, Kaaber S: Hypoalgesic effect of EMLA and lidocaine gel applied on human oral mucosa: quantitative evaluation by sensory and pain thresholds to argon laser stimulation. Anesth Prog 1992; 39: 4-8.

32. Holst A, Evers H: Experimental studies of new topical anaesthetics on the oral mucosa. Swed Dent J 1985; 9: 185-191.

33. Vickers ER, Punnia-Moorthy A: A clinical evaluation of three topical anaesthetic agents. Aust Dental J 1992; 37: 266-270.

34. Ljunghall K, Lillieborg S: Local anaesthesia with a lidocaine/prilocaine cream (EMLA) for cautery of condylomata acuminata on the vulval mucosa. The effect of timing of application of the cream. Acta Derm Venereol 1989; 69: 362-365.

35. Hallen A, Ljunghall K, Wallin J: Topical anaesthesia with local anaesthetic (lidocaine and prilocaine, EMLA) cream for cautery of genital warts. Genitourin Med 1987; 63: 316-319.

36. Amdisen A, Glud V: No influence from topical application of EMLA cream before blood sampling on routine clinical chemistry and haematology measurements. Eur J Clin Pharmacol 1991; 41: 619-620.

37. Juhlin L, Evers H, Broberg F: Inhibition of hyperhidrosis by topical application of a local anesthetic composition. Acta Derm Venereol (Stockholm) 1979; 59: 556-559.

38. Shuttleworth D, Hill S, Marks R, Connelly DM: Relief of experimentally induced pruritus with a novel eutectic mixture of local anaesthetic agents. Br J Dermatol 1988; 119: 535-540.

39. Stow PJ, Glynn CJ, Minor B: EMLA cream in the treatment of postherpetic neuralgia. Efficacy and pharmacokinetic profile. Pain 1989; 39: 301-305.

40. Ohlsén L, Evers H, Segerström K, Hagelqvist E, Graffman S: Local anaesthetics modifying the dermal response of irradiation. Acta Oncol 1987; 6: 467-476.

41. Ritchie JM, Greene NM: Local anesthetics. In: The Pharmacological Basis of Therapeutics. Gilman AG, Goodman LS, Rall TW, Murad F, eds. Macmillan, New York. 1985; 303-321.

42. Juhlin L, Hägglund G, Evers H: Absorption of lidocaine and prilocaine after application of a eutectic mixture of local anesthetics (EMLA) on normal and diseased skin. Acta Derm Venereol 1989; 69: 18-22.

43. Holm J, Andrén B, Grafford K: Pain control in the surgical debridement of leg ulcers by the use of a topical lidocaine-prilocaine cream, EMLA. Acta Derm Venereol 1990; 70: 132-136.

44. Pere P, Iizuka T, Rosenberg PH, Lindqvist C: Topical application of 5% eutectic mixture of lignocaine (EMLA) before removal of arch bars. Br J Oral Maxillofacial Surg 1992; 30: 153-156.

45. Nilsson A, Engberg G, Henneberg S, Danielson K, de Verdier CH: Inverse relationship between age-dependent erythrocyte activity of methaemoglobin reductase and prilocaine-induced methaemoglobinemia during infancy. Br J Anaesth 1990; 64: 72-76.

46. Engberg G, Danielson K, Henneberg S, Nilsson A: Plasma concentrations of prilocaine and lidocaine and methaemoglobin formation in infants after epicutaneous application of a 5% lidocaine-prilocaine cream (EMLA). Acta Anaesth Scand 1987; 3: 624-648.

47. Haugstvedt S, Friman AM, Danielson K: Plasma concentrations of lidocaine and prilocaine and analgesic effect after dermal application of EMLA cream 5% for surgical removal of mollusca in children. Z Kinderchir 1990; 45: 148-150.

48. Manner T, Kanto J, Iisalo E, Lindberg R, Viinamäki O, Scheinin M: Reduction of pain at venous cannulation in children with a eutectic mixture of lidocaine and prilocaine (EMLA cream): comparison with

placebo cream and no local premedication. Anaesthesiol Scand 1987; 31: 735-739.

49. Bruguerolle B, Giaufre E, Prat M: Temporal variations in transcutaneous passage of drugs: the exemple of lidocaine in children and in rats. Chronobiol Int 1991; 8: 277-282.

50. Kravitz H, Elegant LD, Kaiser E, Kagan B: Methemoglobin values in premature and mature infants and children. Am J Dis Child 1956; 91: 1-5.

51. Jakobson B, Nilsson A: Methaemoglobinemia associated with a prilocaine-lidocaine cream and trimetoprim-sulphamethoxazole. A case report. Acta Anaesth Scand 1985; 29: 453-455.

52. Frayling IM, Addison GM, Chattergee K: Methaemoglobinemia in children treated with prilocaine-lidocaine cream. Br Med J 1990; 301: 153-154.

53. Anniko M, Schmidt SH: The ototoxic potential of EMLA. Acta Otolaryngol 1988; 105: 255-265.

54. Anniko M, Hellström S, Schmidt SH, Spandow O: Toxic effects on inner ear of noxious agents passing through the round window membrane. Acta Otolaryngol 1988; 57(Suppl 4): 49-56.

55. Bingham B, Hawke M, Halik J: The safety and efficacy of EMLA cream topical anesthesia for myringotomy and ventilation tube insertion. J Otolaryngol 1991; 20: 193-195.

56. Covino BG: Toxicity and systemic effects of local anesthetic agents. In: Local Anesthetics. Strichartz GR, ed. Handbook of Experimental Pharmacology 181. Springer-Verlag, Berlin. 1987; 187-212.

57. Simons FER, Gillespie CA, Simons KJ: Local anesthetic creams and intradermal skin tests. Lancet 1992; 339: 1351-1352.

58. Pipkorn U, Andersson M: Topical dermal anaesthesia inhibits the flare but not the weal response to allergen and histamine in the skin-prick test. Clin Allergy 1987; 17: 307-311.

59. Björkstein B, Jung B, Tågsjö EB, Groth O: Delayed hypersensitivity responses in children after local cutaneous anesthesia. Acta Paediatr Scand 1987; 76: 935-938.

60. Wehle B, Björnström M, Cedgård M, Danielsson K, Ekernäs A, Gutierrez A, Petterson U, Lindholm T: Repeated aplication of EMLA cream 5% for the alleviation of cannulation pain in haemodialysis. Scand J Urol Nephrol 1989; 23: 299-302.

3

Use of EMLA in Infants and Children Undergoing Venipuncture

Gideon Koren

The Hospital for Sick Children
Toronto, Ontario, Canada

Isabelle Robieux

Centro di Riferimento Oncologico—Aviano
Aviano, Italy

Daniel S. Halperin

Hôpital Cantonal Universitaire
Geneva, Switzerland

I. INTRODUCTION

For many years it was assumed that young children suffer less pain than adults, and infants and children have received substantially less analgesia than adults for the same clinical situations [1]. However, it has now been demonstrated that neurochemical systems and pathways known to be associated with pain are functional even in the fetus [2]. Neonates given adequate anesthesia during surgery were shown to be more clinically stable, with fewer postoperative complications, than those given minimal anesthesia; the latter demonstrated a massive stress response during operations [2]. An increasing number of scientists and cinicians have voiced concern over the minimal analgesia provided in the past for pediatric patients.

Although the long-term effects of painful diagnostic or therapeutic procedures on children are unknown [3,4], there is little doubt that pain may affect, in the short term, both the physical and mental well-being of children and their families, their relationship with the medical and nursing team, and their overall attitude toward medical care. It has been hypothesized that factors such as sex, age, ethnic background, frequency of painful stimulus, and duration of illness may all play a role in the perception and recall of pain by children. It may therefore be important to identify a subgroup of children for whom anticipation of pain is high who may benefit the most from provision of analgesia.

By far the most common use for EMLA® cream since its introduction into clinical medicine has been the alleviation of pain associated with venipuncture in children. The psychological impact of needle pain on the hospitalized child is immense, especially in children with chronic illness who need repeated procedures. Indeed, the fear and pain caused by needles are often perceived by pediatric patients as being worse than those caused by the disease for which they are being treated [5], and can make insertion of intravenous needles or catheters a traumatic experience for the child and a difficult and time-consuming task for the physician or nurse. The alleviation of this pain and fear not only helps such patients to accept medical intervention, but also relieves the stress and time involved in calming the patient.

Many studies have been carried out to assess the efficacy of EMLA cream in venipuncture (Table 1). These studies have involved the difficult task of assessing pain in young, sometimes nonverbalizing, patients. A variety of subjective and objective scores have been

Table 1 Studies Examining the Effect of EMLA on Venipuncture Pain in Children and Adults

Author (Ref.)	Age of patient (years)	Outcome of trial
Clarke and Radford [33]	1–14	$n = 15$. Pain scores with EMLA statistically lower than for placebo (VAS and VRS).
Cooper et al. [34]	3–13	$n = 40$. Pain scores with EMLA statistically lower than for placebo (four assessment methods).
De-Jong et al. [35]	4–12	$n = 64$. Efficacy of EMLA similar to that of ethyl-chloride spray (VAS and VRS).
Dohlwitz and Uppfeldt [36]	4–16	$n = 110$. Pain scores with EMLA statistically lower than for placebo, for all application times (20–75 minutes) (VAS).
Ehrenstrom-Reiz et al. [37]	6–15	$n = 60$. Pain scores with EMLA statistically lower than for placebo.
Gunawardene and Davenport [38]	27–68	$n = 100$. Pain lower with EMLA plus glyceryl trinitrate than with either agent alone or placebo.
Hallen et al. [6]	4–15	$n = 31$. Pain scores lower than (90%) or equal to (10%) placebo.
Halperin et al. [10]	6–12	$n = 18$. Pain scores with EMLA statistically lower than for placebo (VAS).
Hopkins et al. [9]	1–6	$n = 111$. Pain scores with EMLA statistically lower than for placebo (VAS, VRS from observer).
Joyce et al. [39]	5–12	$n = 96$, stratified for age, sex and diagnosis. Pain scores with EMLA statistically lower than for placebo (VAS from child, investigator and nurse)

(Continued)

Table 1 (Continued)

Author (Ref.)	Age of patient (years)	Outcome of trial
Koren [40]	Adults	$n = 6$. Pain scores with EMLA statistically lower than for placebo (VAS, cross-over study).
Kurien et al. [41]	0.08–4	$n = 55$. Pain scores with EMLA statistically lower than for placebo (VRS from observer).
Maddi et al. [42]	Adults	Pain scores with EMLA statistically lower than with placebo for application times longer than 45 minutes.
Manner et al. [8]	4–10	$n = 58$. Pain scores with EMLA statistically lower than for placebo or no treatment (VAS).
Maunuskela and Korpela [7]	4–10	$n = 60$. Pain scores with EMLA statistically lower than for placebo (VRS and visual scale). No difference for "face" scale.
Moller [43]	8–17	$n = 51$. Pain scores with EMLA statistically lower than for placebo (VRS).
Robieux et al. [25]	0.25–3	$n = 58$. Pain scores similar for EMLA and placebo, unless values adjusted for degree of difficulty of needle insertion (BPS, VAS from observer).
Sims [44]	13–15	$n = 100$. "Thick" layer of EMLA is more effective than a "thin" layer (VRS).
Soliman et al. [45]	7–12	$n = 42$. Efficacy of EMLA similar to that of lidocaine infiltration (VAS from child, investigator and observer).
Wig and Johl [46]	1.5–10	$n = 75$. EMLA more effective than placebo.

utilized, including behavioral and physiological alterations, in an attempt to demonstrate alleviation of pain.

Studies involving self-reporting children and adults generally use well-established visual analog scales or verbal rating scores; EMLA cream has been shown to be an effective analgesic for venipuncture in such studies [6–13]. Measurement of pain in nonverbalizing infants and toddlers is a more complex task, requiring reliable and reproducible methods for assessing pain experienced by others. However, the clearly defined pain stimulus of venipuncture, which can be traced accurately in terms of its time of infliction and may be repeated for routine care in the same infant, facilitates assessment of analgesic efficacy in this indication.

This chapter reviews the studies conducted to assess the efficacy of EMLA cream in pediatric patients undergoing venipuncture, concentrating on the few that have been conducted in nonverbalizing infants and toddlers. It should be noted that the international recommended minimum age of 3 months for the use of EMLA cream has been adopted in many countries, but the minimum age in some countries does differ, generally within the range of 1 to 6 months.

II. NONVERBALIZING INFANTS AND TODDLERS

The physiological markers traditionally associated with pain or nociceptive activity in nonverbalizing infants include:

> Changes in cardiovascular variables such as heart rate and blood pressure [14]
> Decreased oxygenation [15]
> Increased palmar sweating [16]
> Hormonal and metabolic changes [2]

The behavioral correlates of the pain experience in neonates include:

> Distinct facial expressions [17]
> Distinct cry patterns, including the absence of crying [18–20]
> Alterations in more complex behavior as well as sleep-wake cycles [18,21,22]

Table 2 Behavioral Pain Score

Behavior to observe	Score (total 0–8)
Facial expression	
Positive, i.e. smiling	0
Neutral	1
Negative, i.e. grimace	2
Cry	
Laughing or giggling	0
Not crying	1
Moaning	2
Full-lunged cry or sobbing	3
Movements	
Usual activities, e.g. in playing	0
Neutral, not moving	1
Attempt to withdraw limb	2
Complex agitation involving head, other limbs	3

Source: Modified from Refs. 23 and 24.

Several behavioral pain scales (BPS) have been developed based on observations of these factors. A scale modified from the Children's Hospital of Eastern Ontario Pain Scale (CHEOPS) by McGrath et al. [23,24] is described in Table 2.

A. Clinical Studies

Study 1

Robieux et al. [25] studied 58 chronically ill children, aged between 3 and 36 months, all of whom had previously undergone venipuncture. Forty-one children were included in a double-blind, cross-over study with EMLA and placebo creams administered in random order, allowing 1 day to 1 month between applications. The remaining children received a single cream only (EMLA or placebo) and did not participate in the cross-over arm of the study.

The EMLA or placebo cream (2 g) was applied to the intended site of venipuncture and left in situ under a Tegaderm® dressing for

Table 3 Mean Change in Behavioral Pain
Score (BPS) in Different Age Groups

	Change in BPS	
Age group (months)	EMLA	Placebo
3–6	1.9	2.1
10–23	1.8	2.9
24–36	0.7	1.4
All ages	1.5[a]	2[a]

[a] $p < 0.01$, Wilcoxon signed rank test.

at least 45 minutes. Venipuncture was then carried out, and the difficulty of the procedure recorded on a 4-point scale, from insertion at first attempt to failure of two or more attempts.

Pain was scored using visual analog scales (VAS) of 0 (no pain) to 100 (maximum pain) on which the investigators, nurses, and parents estimated the degree of pain suffered by the infant. The BPS described in Table 2 [23,24] was used for the patient. Behavior and cry were monitored throughout by video and sound level meter; blood pressure and pulse were recorded 1 minute before, during, and 5 minutes after the procedure.

The BPS results are shown in Table 3. An increase in BPS suggests greater pain; therefore little or no increase generally signifies effective analgesia. This does not apply in cases in which the baseline BPS is high, as was observed in 25% of the patients in this study. In 25 patients with a low baseline BPS who participated in the cross-over study, the mean increase in BPS was similar for EMLA cream and placebo. The efficacy appeared to depend on the age of the patient; in younger infants (age < 9 months) there was little difference between EMLA and placebo, whereas in older patients (24 to 36 months), the increase in BPS with placebo was twice that observed with EMLA cream.

The VAS results are shown in Table 4. If the needle insertion was successful on the first attempt, and the pain experienced was mild,

Table 4 Visual Analog Scale (VAS)
Mean and Standard Deviation

Observer	EMLA	Placebo
Investigator	36 ± 25	44 ± 26
Nurse	29 ± 26	38 ± 25
Parent	37 ± 31	43 ± 27

then the efficacy of EMLA cream was easily demonstrated. However, the reported VAS values correlated strongly with the scores for difficulty of venipuncture, which were similar for both placebo- and EMLA-treated groups. When the VAS values were adjusted by a factor correcting for difficulty of puncture, the calculated scores were lower in the EMLA-treated group than in the placebo group.

There were no statistically significant differences between the two groups for changes in heart rate or systolic and diastolic blood pressure. The peak cry intensity increased during puncture in 58% of cases and decreased or remained unchanged in 42%. There was no significant difference between the placebo and EMLA-treated groups.

As EMLA cream has been associated with methemoglobinemia [26,27]; methemoglobin analyses were carried out in some cases. The methemoglobin level was higher than normal (11.3 g/L) in one placebo-treated patient, but the mean levels for each arm of the trial were normal and were similar for EMLA cream and placebo. Local reactions, observed after both placebo and EMLA treatment, included four cases of skin blanching and six cases of redness at the site of the occlusive dressing adhesive.

Study 2

Hopkins et al. evaluated EMLA cream in young children and infants in a randomized, placebo-controlled, double-blind study completed by 111 children, aged 1 to 5 years, who required venipuncture for the induction of general anesthesia [9]. Seventy-five children received EMLA cream and 36 received a placebo cream. Approximately one-third of the patients in each group were premedicated.

Pain was assessed by a single observer on a 100 mm VAS, in which 0 represented no pain and 100 severe pain, and on a 4-point verbal rating scale consisting of the following four categories: (1) no reaction: no whimpering, grimacing, or reflex movement; (2) slight pain: whimpering, grimacing, minor reflex movement; (3) moderate pain: continual whimpering, grimacing, reflex movement; and (4) severe pain: loud crying, intense reflex movement. The EMLA-treated group had significantly lower pain ratings on both the VAS and the verbal scale. Within each group, patients who received premedication had lower ratings than those who did not. No correlation was found between condition on arrival, application time of EMLA cream, and VAS.

Side effects of EMLA treatment were mild local pallor in 36 patients, moderate local pallor in six patients, and erythema in four patients. These reactions disappeared within 1 hour.

The investigators concluded that the use of EMLA cream should be standard clinical practice for all children undergoing venipuncture. Indeed, pretreatment with EMLA cream is now standard practice before venipuncture in children at the Royal Liverpool Children's Hospital in the United Kingdom, where this study was conducted.

Study 3

Kurien et al. [28] carried out a double-blind, parallel-group study in Oriental infants, to assess whether EMLA cream was effective in children of this race and skin color. Twenty-eight children (median age 30 months) were given placebo cream and 27 (median age 24 months) were treated with EMLA cream at least 1 hour prior to venipuncture. Pain was rated for all children by a single observer, using a 3-point scale of no pain, slight pain, or severe pain.

The results demonstrated significantly lower pain scores with EMLA cream than with placebo, irrespective of the area of insertion of the needle (hand, arm, or cubital fossa). Blanching was not observed, possibly because the darker skin of the Oriental children concealed this phenomenon. The report noted the difficulty of assessing pain in infants, but pointed out that the randomized, double-blind nature of the trial and assessment of pain by a single observer helped to control bias.

B.   Methodological Considerations

The above studies demonstrate the superiority of EMLA cream over placebo in alleviating pain associated with venipuncture; however, the results are not as clearly defined as those obtained with older (verbalizing) children and adults [6–13]. The mean BPS increased on venipuncture for both placebo- and EMLA-treated patients, and although the mean increase with EMLA cream was statistically lower, in certain infants (especially those less than 9 months old) the BPS with EMLA cream were higher than those with placebo.

Some data suggest that the BPS may not be an appropriate measure to assess acute pain in infants. For example, the motor behavior of neonates during a heel-prick was monitored by Booth and McGrath [29]. The preparation phases of the process were found to be associated with increased distress body movements, and the actual puncture yielded little further increase in movement. Thus, as distress symptoms occur before pain is inflicted, body movements at the time of the infliction of pain would not give a reliable indication of the amount of pain felt, particularly in infants with prior experience of a procedure. In the study by Robieux et al. [25], baseline BPS were high in 25% of patients, probably reflecting anxiety through previous experience of venipuncture.

The use of VAS has been validated as an appropriate way to assess pain in self-reporting patients [30]; indeed, patients as young as 4 years old are able to use VAS provided they perceive differences in pain intensity as a continuum. Although several studies have relied on VAS completed by observers, based on what they have seen, heard, or felt, it is more difficult to judge the validity of these scores. The VAS scores reported depend on the observer's own experiences of pain and on any knowledge of the child's usual behavior. For example, the observer may consider that a difficult/unsuccessful venipuncture attempt is painful, and score accordingly. However, the higher VAS scores seen with difficult procedures [25] may be a true reflection of the lower efficacy of EMLA cream when the venipuncture needle is moved into deeper tissues.

An additional problem with very young children is lack of knowledge of how they experience pain. Pain may be experienced as a dose-response effect, in which a greater stimulus produces an increased response or, alternatively, young children may have a threshold pain level at which full distress response behavior is elicited. As the VAS and BPS rely on patients' perceiving pain as a continuum, these scores would have limited meaning in the case of a pain threshold.

The measurements of heart rate and blood pressure made by Robieux et al. [25] did not provide any additional information over that supplied by the BPS. In infants who showed no distress behavior there were no changes in heart rate and blood pressure. Heart rate and blood pressure increased in only about half of the infants for whom distress behavior was obvious. The peak intensity of cry also appeared to be a poor predictor of pain relief.

Analgesia should be optimally evaluated by self-reporting patients who experience the painful procedure themselves. Such assessment is not possible with infants (who, by the Latin definition of the term, are "not speaking"), and adults may lack the ability to interpret correctly their rich, nonverbal language used to express pain. The old attitude that young children suffer less pain than adults may have resulted from this inability of observers to distinguish between stress and pain responses in infants. The efficacy of EMLA cream demonstrated by the above studies suggests that infants do, in fact, experience pain and can benefit from analgesic drugs, as do older children and adults in similar circumstances.

C. Safety of EMLA

To date, all studies have indicated that the use of EMLA cream in infants over 3 months of age is not associated with any local or systemic adverse effects when applied on a limited skin area for less than 90 minutes. Skin absorption of drugs is known to be enhanced in infants, and can potentially lead to systemic toxicity [27,31,32]. As discussed in Chapter 2, the prilocaine component of EMLA cream is metabolized to compounds capable of inducing the formation of methemoglobin [27]. This problem is likely to occur only in infants of less than 3 months old, in whom the activity of the methemoglobin reduction pathway is lower than in adults. However, with the normal conditions of use associated with venipuncture reported by

Robieux et al. [25], the EMLA group had methemoglobin levels similar to those of the placebo group, even in the youngest infants. This indicates that systemic absorption of the anesthetics was clinically insignificant.

III. VERBALIZING CHILDREN

In contrast to studies with infants and toddlers, there are many published studies that have compared EMLA cream to placebo and/or to other modes of skin anesthesia (e.g. ethyl chloride spray, lidocaine infiltration) in verbalizing children of all ages or in adults. These studies are almost invariably double-blind and randomized; most are placebo-controlled and are either parallel or cross-over (i.e. the same patient received both EMLA and placebo creams) in design. Many of the studies investigate the effect of application time on the efficacy of EMLA cream.

Table 1 summarizes the main outcomes of trials conducted with EMLA cream in children and adults. The following examples, which are discussed in greater detail, highlight some of the issues addressed by such trials.

A. Clinical Studies

Study 1

Halperin et al. [10] carried out a randomized, double-blind, placebo-controlled study involving 18 children, aged 6 to 12 years, who were receiving venipuncture for administration of chemotherapy. EMLA or placebo cream (2 g) was applied to the dorsum of the hand and covered with an occlusive dressing (Tegaderm®) for 30 to 175 minutes. The dressing and cream were removed 1 to 20 minutes before the puncture, and any local reactions such as pallor, erythema, or edema noted. After venipuncture, pain was scored by the children using a 10 cm visual analog scale (VAS) ranging from 0 (no sensation) to 10 (worst imaginable pain).

The EMLA and placebo groups were well matched in terms of age, sex, duration of cream application, and time lag between removal of cream and venipuncture. The mean pain score for the EMLA group (2.8 ± 2.4) was statistically lower than that for the placebo group (6.8 ± 2.1) ($p < 0.01$). The efficacy of EMLA cream depended on the application time of the cream. The mean pain score for children treated with EMLA cream for 30 to 50 minutes was 4.7, compared with a score of 1.8 for those treated for longer than 60 minutes ($p < 0.05$).

The use of VAS has recently been validated in young children. Good correlation with behavioral assessments is shown provided that the patient is capable of comprehending pain as a graduated phenomenon. During a preliminary teaching session on the VAS, all children in this study [10] were able to understand the concept of pain and of pain severity.

Study 2

Hallén et al. conducted a placebo-controlled, cross-over trial in 31 adult subjects undergoing a voluntary occupational health investigation. Eight venous blood samples were required from each subject; five were taken after application of EMLA cream and three after application of placebo. EMLA or placebo cream (2 g) was applied under an occlusive dressing to the cubital fossa or dorsum of the hand for 1 hour. On removal of the cream, any local reactions were noted, and then venipuncture was carried out immediately. Pain was rated by the subjects using a VAS ranging from 0 (no pain) to 100 (painful).

EMLA cream was superior to placebo in all but three subjects, who rated EMLA and placebo as equal. The scores after application of EMLA cream tended to cluster around the "no pain" end of the scale, whereas those for placebo were scattered over the whole range. The mean pain score for EMLA was significantly lower ($p < 0.001$) than that for placebo. Local reactions, such as pallor and erythema, were mild and transient, and were equally distributed between the EMLA and placebo treatments.

Study 3

Maunuksela and Korpela [7] compared EMLA cream with placebo in a randomized double-blind study involving 60 children aged 4 to 10 years who were due to undergo cannulation for the induction of general anesthesia. EMLA or placebo cream (2 g) was applied for at least 60 minutes. Pain was assessed by the children using two different pictorial scales, one depicting smiling and crying faces and one showing a sloping colored scale (marked 0 to 50). In addition, pain was rated by both the anesthetist and the patients using a 4-point verbal rating scale (VRS). Preoperative tests demonstrated that the children were able to use the scales correctly.

There was a significant difference between the EMLA cream and the placebo scores for verbal ratings given by both the anesthetist and the patients. The anesthetist rated the efficacy of EMLA cream slightly higher than the patients. When the patients' VRS scores were analyzed according to the childrens' age, scores with EMLA cream were significantly lower than placebo scores for the 7- to 10-year-olds, but no significant difference was detected in the 4- to 6-year-old age group. This was thought to be due to the attitude of the older children, who understood the medical procedure more clearly and were consequently less emotional and distressed.

The pain assessments made using the visual colored scale were statistically lower for the EMLA group than the placebo group (12.4 and 23.5, respectively; $p < 0.05$), but those obtained using the "face" scale did not show any statistical difference between the two groups.

IV. CONCLUSION

All studies conducted in verbalizing children and adults have shown a clinically and/or statistically significant decrease in pain with EMLA cream. Different centers in many countries have reported overwhelmingly the effectiveness of EMLA cream for venipuncture. Indeed, there are few other instances in which a new therapeutic agent in pediatric medicine has yielded such unanimous agreement over its efficacy. This record is even more impressive when consideration is given to the negligible risk of serious adverse reactions. Side effects are, in general, mild and transient; severe effects are confined mainly to children allergic to amide anesthetics.

Studies of EMLA cream use in pediatric venipuncture constitute the largest human experience with this product. The homogeneity of the results in terms of efficacy are striking, even with young, non-verbalizing infants. At present it seems unnecessary, and probably unethical, to undertake further studies on the efficacy of EMLA cream for venipuncture, as EMLA has been proven superior to placebo in all 20 of the blinded trials reviewed here.

Ethical considerations should guarantee that all children over 3 months of age (the international recommended minimum age for use) undergoing venipuncture are offered EMLA treatment. Once the safety profile of EMLA has been fully assessed in infants aged under 3 months, then the use of EMLA cream might be extended to this age group.

REFERENCES

1. Schechter NL: The undertreatment of pain in children: an overview. Ped Clin North Am 1989; 36(4): 781-94.
2. Anand KJS, Phil D, Hickey PR: Pain and its effects in the human neonate and fetus. N Engl J Med 1987; 317: 1321-1329.
3. Schechter NL, Allen DA, Hanson K: Status of pediatric pain control: a comparison of hospital analgesic usage in children and adults. Pediatrics 1986; 77: 11-15.
4. Stevens B, Hunsberger M, Browne G: Pain in children: theoretical, research, and practice dilemmas. J Pediatr Nurs 1987; 2: 154-166.
5. Rice LJ: Needle phobia: an anesthesiologist's perspective. J Pediatr 1993; 122: S9-S13.
6. Hallen B, Carlsson P, Uppfeldt A. Clinical study of a lidocaine-prilocaine cream to relieve the pain of venipuncture. Br J Anaesth 1985; 57: 326-328.
7. Maunuskela EL, Korpela R: Double-blind evaluation of lidocaine-prilocaine cream (EMLA) in children. Br J Anaesth 1986; 58: 1242-1245.
8. Manner T, Kanto J, Lindbergh R, Viinamaki O, Schein M: Reduction of pain at venous cannulation in children with a eutectic mixture of lidocaine and prilocaine (EMLA) cream: comparison with placebo cream and no local premedication. Acta Anesthesiol Scand 1987; 31: 735-739.
9. Hopkins CS, Buckley CJ, Bush GH: Pain-free injection in infants. Anaesthesia 1988; 43: 198-201.

10. Halperin DL, Koren G, Attias D, Pellegrini E, Greenberg M, Wyss M: Topical skin anesthesia for venous, subcutaneous drug reservoir and lumbar punctures in children. Pediatrics 1989; 84: 281-284.

11. Kapelushnik J, Koren G, Solh H, Greenberg M, Levert DeVeber: Evaluating the efficacy of EMLA in alleviating pain associated with lumbar puncture: comparison of open and double blinded protocols in children. Pain 1990; 42: 31-34.

12. Juhlin L, Evers H, Broberg F: A lidocaine-prilocaine cream for superficial skin surgery and painful lesions. Acta Derm Venerol 1980; 60: 544-546.

13. Arendt-Nielsen L, Bjerring P: Laser induced pain for evaluation of local analgesia: a comparison of topical application (EMLA) and local injection (lidocaine). Anesth Analg 1988; 67: 115-123.

14. Williamson PS, Williamson ML: Physiological stress reduction by a local anesthetic during newborn circumcision. Pediatrics 1983; 71: 36-40.

15. Rawlings DJ, Miller PA, Engel RR: The effect of circumcision on transcutaneous pO_2 in term infants. Am J Dis Child 1980; 134: 676-678.

16. Harpin VA, Rutter N: Development of emotional sweating in the newborn infant. Arch Dis Child 1982; 57: 691-695.

17. Grunau RVE, Johnston CC, Craig KD: Neonatal facial and cry responses to invasive and non-invasive procedures. Pain 1990; 42: 295-305.

18. Emde RN, Harmon RJ, Metcalf D et al: Stress and neonatal sleep. Psychosom Med 1971; 33: 491-497.

19. Porter FL, Miller RH, Marshall RE: Neonatal pain cries: Effect of circumcision on acoustic features and perceived urgency. Child Dev 1986; 57: 790-802.

20. Pacifiers, passive behaviour, and pain (editorial). Lancet 1992; 339: 275-276.

21. Marshall RE, Stratton WC, Moore JA, Boxerman SB: Circumcision. I: Effects upon newborn behaviour. Infant Behav Dev 1980; 3: 1-14.

22. Marshall RE, Porter FL, Rogers AG, Moore JA, Anderson B, Boxerman SB: Circumcision. II: Effects upon mother-infant interaction. Early Human Dev 1982; 7: 367-374.

23. McGrath P: An assessment of children's pain: a review of behavioral, physiological and direct scaling techniques. Pain 1987; 31: 147-176.

24. McGrath PJ, Johnson G, Goodman JT et al: The children of Eastern Ontario Pain Scale (CHEOPS): a behavioral scale for rating postoperative pain in children. In: Advances in Pain Research and Therapy. Fields HL, Dubner R, Cervero F (eds). New York, Raven Press. 1985; 9: 395-402.

25. Robieux I, Kumar R, Radhakrishnan S, Koren G: Assessing pain and analgesia with a lidocaine-prilocaine emulsion in infants and toddlers during venipuncture. J Pediatr 1991; 118: 971-973.

26. Gosselin RE, Hodge HC, Smith RP: In: Clinical Toxicology of Commercial Products. Vol III. Baltimore, Williams & Wilkins. 1984; 31-35, 314-319.

27. Jakobson B, Nilson A: Methemoglobinemia associated with a prilocaine-lidocaine cream and trimethopim-sulfamethoxazole. A case report. Acta Anesthesiol Scand. 1985; 29: 453-455.

28. Kurien L, Kollberg H, Uppfeldt A: Venepuncture pain can be reduced. J Trop Med Hyg 1985; 88: 397-399.

29. Booth JC, McGrath PA, Brigham M, Frewen TC, Whitthall S: Pain in infants: distress response to painful stimuli. Canadian and American Pain Societies, Toronto, Canada. 1988; Abstract 66.

30. Scott J, Huskinsson EC: Graphic representation of pain. Pain 1976; 2: 175-184.

31. Mofenson HC, Caraccio TR: Lidocaine toxicity from topical mucosal application. Clin Pediatr 1983; 22: 190-192.

32. Sundaram MB: Seizures after intraurethral instillation of lidocaine. Can Med Assoc J 1987; 137: 219-220.

33. Clarke S, Radford M: Topical anesthesia for venipuncture. Arch Dis Child 1986; 61: 1132-1134.

34. Cooper CM, Gerrish SP, Hardwick M, Kay R: EMLA cream reduces the pain of venipuncture in children. Eur J Anaesth 1987; 4: 441-448.

35. de Jong PC, Verburg MP, Lillieborg S: EMLA® cream versus ethylchloride spray: a comparison of the analgesic efficacy in children. Eur J Anaesth 1990; 7: 473-481.

36. Dohlwitz A, Uppfeldt A: Schmerzlinderung bei Venenpukion. Applikation und Wirksamkeit einer Lidocain-Prilocain-Creme. Anaesthesist 1985; 34: 355-358.

37. Ehrenstrom Reiz GME, Reiz SLA: EMLA: a eutectic mixture of local anaesthetics for topical anaesthesia. Acta Anaesth Scand 1982; 26: 596-598.

38. Gunawardene RD, Davenport HT: Local application of EMLA and glyceryl trinitrate ointment before venipuncture. Anaesthesia 1990; 45: 52-54.

39. Joyce TH, Skjonsby BS, Taylor BD, Morrow DH, Hess KR: Dermal anesthesia using a eutectic mixture of lidocaine and prilocaine (EMLA) for venipuncture in children. Pain Digest 1992; 2: 137-141.

40. Koren G: Topical skin anesthesia. In: Clinics in Dermatology. Shear N (ed). 1989; 7: 136-141.

41. Kurien L, Kollberg H, Uppfeldt A: Venipuncture pain can be reduced. J Trop Med Hyg 1985; 88: 397-399.

42. Maddi R, Horrow JC, Mark JB, Conception M, Murray E: Evaluation of a new cutaneous topical anesthesia preparation. RegiAnesth 1990; 15: 109-112.

43. Moller C: A lignocaine-prilocaine cream reduces venipuncture pain. Uppsala J Med Sci 1985; 90: 293-398.

44. Sims C: Thickly and thinly applied lignocaine-prilocaine cream prior to venipuncture in children. Anaesth Int Care 1991; 19: 343-345.

45. Soliman IE, Broadman LM, Hannallah RS, McGill WA: Comparison of the analgesic effects of EMLA (eutectic mixture of local anesthetics) to intradermal lidocaine infiltration prior to venous cannulation in un-premedicated children. Anesthesiology 1988; 68: 804-806.

46. Wig J, Johl KS: Our experience with EMLA cream (for painless venous cannulation in children). Ind J Physiol Pharmac 1990; 34: 130-132.

4

Topical Skin Anesthesia for Subcutaneous Drug Reservoir and Lumbar Punctures in Children

Gideon Koren

The Hospital for Sick Children
Toronto, Ontario, Canada

Daniel S. Halperin and Marinette Wyss

Hôpital Cantonal Universitaire
Geneva, Switzerland

Joseph Kapelushnik

Rothschild Hospital
Haifa, Israel

I. INTRODUCTION

The treatment of leukemia in children requires that lumbar punctures be repeated periodically, to rule out central nervous system involvement and to administer chemotherapy. Likewise, cancer treatment requires repeated access to the venous blood to allow intravenous therapy and monitor for response and adverse effects. Unfortunately, in many youngsters the task of finding a suitable superficial vein becomes a major problem; therefore, subcutaneous drug reservoirs are surgically inserted in the subclavicular areas to allow repeated access to venous blood through the chest skin.

Both these types of needle punctures are painful, eliciting immense anxiety in pediatric patients and their parents, and therefore posing stress on pediatricians who have to perform the procedure [1,2]. As discussed in Chapter 3, any means of alleviating the pain associated with such procedures is likely to increase the well-being of the children (and their parents and health care workers), the quality of their care, and, indeed, the acceptability of their treatment: objectives that are especially important in children already suffering from a debilitating disease such as cancer.

This chapter reviews the efficacy of EMLA® cream in reducing the pain associated with lumbar punctures and injections through subcutaneous drug reservoirs. Methodological issues important in evaluating skin anesthesia in children, such as the value of carrying out blinded studies, are also considered. Only a few studies have been carried out with EMLA cream in these indications; those located to date were conducted in children suffering from malignant diseases who had been enrolled in various chemotherapy protocols for at least 6 months. None of the children had received analgesia or sedation prior to the studies.

II. SUBCUTANEOUS DRUG RESERVOIRS

Only one study of the use of EMLA cream in relieving pain from subcutaneous drug reservoirs has been reported. Halperin et al. [3] studied eight children (6 to 15 years old) who underwent injections through a subclavicular drug reservoir, without premedication. All patients had previous experience of punctures through a reservoir for administration of chemotherapy. The randomized, double-blind, cross-over study involved application of EMLA or placebo cream for

Table 1 Comparison of Pain Scores in EMLA- and Placebo-Treated Children Undergoing Subcutaneous Drug Reservoir Puncture

	EMLA	Placebo
Number of patients	8	
Age (years)		
Median	10.7	
Range	6.1–15.1	
Duration of cream application (min)		
Mean	92	89
Range	60–175	68–165
Time from removal of cream to venipuncture (min)		
Mean	4.5	3.6
Range	1–10	1–5
Pain score		
Mean (± SD)	1.2 (± 1.8)[a]	3.9 (± 2.2)[a]
Range	0–5	0–7

[a] Significant difference between treatment groups $p < 0.004$ (Wilcoxon signed-rank test).

approximately 60 minutes. The time interval between the cross-over arms of the study was between 1 and 4 weeks in each patient. The children rated pain experienced during the procedure using a visual analog scale (VAS) in which 0 denoted no pain and 10 denoted maximum possible pain.

Mean pain scores are given in Table 1. There was a significant difference between the EMLA and placebo scores, and seven of eight children rated EMLA cream superior to the placebo. The duration of cream application was similar for EMLA and the placebo, as was the mean time interval between wiping off the cream and puncture (Table 1).

Since the completion of this study, EMLA cream is routinely offered in Toronto and Geneva for children with cancer undergoing injection into a subcutaneous drug reservoir.

III. LUMBAR PUNCTURE

A. Clinical Studies

Two studies investigating the use of EMLA cream during lumbar puncture have been reported. In the first, Halperin et al. [3] studied 14 children aged 5.5 to 15 years who were undergoing lumbar punctures at the time of intrathecal chemotherapy. EMLA or placebo creams were applied for 1 hour. The cross-over study design involved the same investigator performing both the EMLA and the placebo punctures, with an interval between the two arms of the study of 1 to 6 weeks for each patient. Ten of the patients had previous experience of lumbar puncture, but four had never experienced the procedure prior to entry into the study.

Mean pain scores, duration of cream application, and interval between removal of the cream and puncture are given in Table 2. There was a significant difference between the EMLA and placebo scores, and EMLA cream was preferred by 12 of the 14 children. Pain scores for the subgroups who had or had not experienced previous lumbar punctures were not statistically different, suggesting that prior knowledge of the procedure had no influence on pain evaluation.

The second study was carried out by Kapelushnik et al. [4], who studied the effect of blinding on the assessment of the analgesic effect of EMLA cream in two groups of children undergoing lumbar puncture. Eighteen children with acute lymphoblastic leukemia participated in an open, cross-over comparison of EMLA cream vs. no treatment. For the EMLA arm of this trial, EMLA cream (2 g) was applied at the intended site of puncture and covered with an occlusive adhesive dressing (Tegaderm®) for 45 to 60 minutes. The assessment of pain associated with a puncture performed without local anaesthesia was randomly carried out 1 month either before or after the EMLA puncture. Following each lumbar puncture, researchers interviewed the observing parents, the nurse who helped during the procedure, and the children. A 100 mm visual analog scale (VAS) was used for measuring pain, ranging from a score of 0 for no pain to 5 for the worst imaginable pain.

Kapelushnik et al. [4] also compared EMLA cream to placebo cream in a cross-over, double-blind trial. Ten children were randomized to receive first either EMLA or placebo cream, which was applied

Table 2 Comparison of Pain Scores in EMLA- and Placebo-Treated Children Undergoing Lumbar Puncture

	EMLA	Placebo
Number of patients	14	
Age (years)		
Median	9.1	
Range	5.5–15.3	
Duration of cream application (min)		
Mean	73	73
Range	60–100	65–90
Time from removal of cream to venipuncture (min)		
Mean	4.1	4.6
Range	2–8	1–20
Pain score		
Mean (± SD)	1.9 (± 1.9)[a]	5.6 (± 3.0)[a]
Range	0–6	0–10

[a] Significant difference between treatment groups $p < 0.01$ (Wilcoxon signed-rank test).

using the procedure described above. The interval between cross-over studies was 4 to 8 weeks. In addition to the VAS described above, children graded pain by using a second 5-point VAS showing facial expressions ranging from smiling (no pain) to crying (maximal pain). Nurses' scores were also recorded using the "face" analog.

The population characteristics and results from both the open and the blinded trials are given in Table 3. In the open trial, there was a statistically significant difference ($p < 0.0005$) between the EMLA and no-treatment scores of the children, parents, and nurses (see Table 3). None of the children rated no treatment as being better than EMLA cream, 16 reported pain relief with EMLA cream, and only two did not detect a difference. However, parents did not detect a difference between EMLA cream and no treatment in six cases, and in five cases the nurses did not detect any differences.

There were also significant differences between the EMLA and placebo scores in the double-blind part of the trial, for both the

Table 3 Comparison of Pain Scores in Blinded and Unblinded Trials with EMLA in Children Undergoing Lumbar Puncture

	Open trial	Blinded trial	
Number of patients	18	10	
Age: mean ± SD (range)	9.2 ± 3.9 (5–15)	6.1 ± 2.1 (4.5–11)	
Sex (male:female)	5:13	8:2	
Application times (min)	45–60	EMLA: 45–100 (mean 77.8 ± 23) Placebo:45–120 (mean 84.5 ± 32)	

	Pain score (scale = 0–5)		Statistical difference
	EMLA	Control	
Unblinded (control = no treatment)			
Child (VAS)	1.7 ± 0.83	2.6 ± 0.6	$p < 0.0005$
Parent (VAS)	1.7 ± 0.9	2.4 ± 0.7	$p < 0.0005$
Nurse (VAS)	1.6 ± 0.8	2.4 ± 0.5	$p < 0.0005$
Blinded (control = placebo cream)			
Child (VAS)	2.0 ± 1.4	3.1 ± 1.0	$p = 0.05$
(face analog scale)	2.9 ± 1.7	3.8 ± 1.2	$p = 0.07$
Nurse (VAS)			
(face analog scale)	2.7 ± 1.1	3.7 ± 0.8	$p < 0.05$

childrens' and the nurses' ratings (see Table 3). There was a significant correlation between the two methods of scoring used by the children (VAS and face analog scale), but no correlation between the face analog scores of the nurses and children. In two of the 10 children, both nurses and children rated the pain experienced with placebo as being lower than that with EMLA cream. These two patients were young children (aged 4.5 and 5 years) who were exposed to EMLA cream for periods shorter than average (45 and 60 minutes). Their scores may support previous studies showing that the ability to report pain as a continuous variable is limited at younger ages [5–7]. In addition, the relationship between time of exposure to EMLA cream and its effectiveness in reducing pain is well documented [7]. The nurses' grading of placebo as being better suggests an incomplete effect of EMLA cream.

Combined results from the blinded and open trials did not show any correlation between a patient's age and the pain scores, and there were no differences between pain scores for boys and girls.

B. Methodological Considerations

The double-blind arm of the trial by Kapelushnik et al [4] revealed significant correlation between scores from two types of VAS recorded by each child. However, there was no correlation between the child's and the nurse-observer's scoring. This suggests that an observer's estimate of pain in nonverbalizing children may be inaccurate. It is often difficult for observers of young children to separate "pain" from "stress" responses, the latter being elicited by anxiety, hunger, and symptoms related to the disease or drug therapy.

The study by Kapelushnik et al. [4] also created a rare and interesting opportunity to evaluate the placebo effect and the impact of blinding in children. While the therapeutic effects of placebo are well known to clinicians caring for children, and double-blind studies utilizing a placebo are the gold standard for clinical trials, little has been done to prove that placebo and blinding are needed in the pediatric age group. Many parents oppose the "deceiving nature" of placebo-controlled drug trials and the ethics of using placebo in nonconsenting individuals are regularly debated [8].

In the open protocol, EMLA cream was found by all patients to be more effective or equal to no treatment. However, in the blinded experiment, EMLA cream was reported to be inferior to placebo in two cases. Although this apparent inferiority of EMLA cream may be explained by the extreme youth of the patients and the shorter application time of EMLA cream, it is important to consider the difference in the results of the open and blinded trials. Both studies suggested favorable effects of EMLA cream, but the blinded study only just reached statistical significance. In open studies, results may be affected not only by the placebo effect but also by physicians' bias, and these results reinforce the need for randomized, placebo-controlled studies involving adequate numbers of children.

IV. CONCLUSION

EMLA cream provided a painless method of application of local anaesthesia (in contrast to lidocaine infiltration, which is often used for lumbar punctures), and it appeared superior to placebo in alleviating pain associated with subcutaneous drug reservoir and lumbar punctures.

REFERENCES

1. Schechter NL, Allen DA, Hanson K: Status of pediatric pain control: a comparison of hospital analgesic usage in children and adults. Pediatrics 1986; 77: 11-15.
2. Stevens B, Hunsberger M, Browne G: Pain in children: theoretical, research, and practice dilemmas. J Pediatr Nurs 1987; 2: 154-166.
3. Halperin DS, Koren G, Attias D, Pellegrini E, Greenberg ML, Wyss M: Topical skin anesthesia for venous, subcutaneous drug reservoir and lumbar punctures in children. Pediatrics 1989; 84: 281-284.
4. Kapelushnik J, Koren G, Solh H, Greenberg M, DeVeber L: Evaluating the efficacy of EMLA in alleviating pain associated with lumbar puncture: comparison of open and double-blinded protocols in children. Pain 1990; 42: 31-34.
5. Beyer JE, Aradine CR: Content validity of an instrument to measure young children's perception of the intensity of their pain. J Pediatr Nurs 1986; 1: 386-395.
6. Elliot CH, Jay SM, Woody P: An observation scale for measuring children's distress during medical procedures. J Pediatr Psychol 1987; 12: 543-551.
7. Maunuksela EL, Olkkola KT, Korpela R: Measurement of pain in children with self reporting and behavioral assessment. Clin Pharmacol Ther 1987; 42: 137-141.
8. Cohen SN: Ethics of drug research in children. In: Pediatric pharmacology. Yaffe SM (ed). Grune & Stratton, New York. 1980; 93-99.

5

Use of EMLA Cream and EMLA Patch in Outpatient Clinics

Gideon Koren, Chrisoula Eliopoulos, Shyam Radhakrishnan, Ram Kumar, and Paul Hwang

The Hospital for Sick Children
Toronto, Ontario, Canada

Isabelle Robieux

Centro di Riferimento Oncologico—Aviano
Aviano, Italy

I. INTRODUCTION

Numerous studies have demonstrated that, in order to achieve effective analgesia, EMLA® cream must be applied to the skin for at least 60 minutes (see Chapter 2). This delay in onset of analgesia is perceived by many as being a major drawback to its use in busy outpatient clinics, where the introduction of a waiting period could affect scheduling. The possibility that using EMLA cream will cause delays in outpatient clinics may lead to physicians dismissing this opportunity of providing pain-free administration of effective analgesia.

To determine whether outpatient clinic schedules would be affected by the waiting period necessary with EMLA cream, the routine delay between admittance and treatment must be assessed. If this delay is longer than 1 hour, it may be possible to use EMLA cream with no additional waiting time and little disruption to normal routine practice. Even if normal waiting times are less than 1 hour, it may be possible for patients (or their parents) to apply EMLA at home, either in the form of a cream under an occlusive dressing or as the new EMLA patch unit-dose package, at an appropriate time before attending the clinic.

This chapter focuses on the feasibility of using EMLA cream in an outpatient setting without disrupting normal routine practice. The likely degree of schedule disruption and the possibility of patients using EMLA cream at home prior to attending outpatient clinics are assessed. Data relating to the EMLA patch, which has a new, unique potential for easy home use, are also reported here.

II. OUTPATIENT CLINICS

Very little published data are available on normal waiting times encountered during standard clinical procedures. One study by Robieux et al. [1] systematically reviewed the routine practice of several outpatient clinics in a large paediatric hospital. Forty children from the Division of Haematology/Oncology and 31 children from the Division of Neurology at The Hospital for Sick Children in Toronto were observed during the course of their visit at these outpatient clinics. The clinics were chosen because many of the visiting patients receive regularly scheduled blood analysis or chemotherapy. In the hematology/oncology clinic, the time of registration for patients scheduled for blood analysis and/or chemotherapy was noted, then each patient was monitored to determine the total period between registration and venipuncture. A similar procedure was used in the neurology clinic, except that the initial time recording was made when patients were first seen by the neurology staff nurse rather than on registration.

In addition to the above clinics, a total of 274 outpatients from the nephrology, gastroenterology, cardiology and rheumatology clinics at The Hospital for Sick Children were studied. Patients attending these clinics were examined by the staff physician prior to the decision to undertake blood analysis. Thus, once the decision for blood analysis was requested by the physician, the only time lag these patients experienced prior to venipuncture was the wait at the phlebotomy station. For patients requiring blood analysis at these clinics, Robieux et al. [1] recorded the period between arrival at the phlebotomy station and the time of venipuncture. The time required by the phlebotomy nurse to choose an appropriate site for venipuncture was also noted for a random set of 20 patients: the mean time was 41.7 ± 39.3 seconds (range 8 to 174 seconds). An average of 1 minute was therefore added to the 60 minutes required for cream application, to yield 61 minutes as the minimum time required at the phlebotomy station for EMLA anesthesia.

A. Hematology/Oncology Clinic

The mean waiting time of patients in the hematology/oncology clinic prior to venipuncture was 131.3 ± 79.5 minutes (range of 10 to 329 minutes), which was statistically longer ($p \leq 0.0005$) than the 60 minutes required for anesthesia [1]. Of the 40 patients observed, only six (15%) underwent venipuncture prior to 60 minutes. Current routine practice at hematology/oncology clinics in most pediatric hospitals requires that patients, after registration at the clinic, proceed to the clinic's own finger-prick station for capillary blood analysis and then wait for consultation with the physician. The majority of the waiting time between registration and venipuncture is required for carrying out tests on the patient's capillary blood sample, which enable the physician to either approve or cancel scheduled blood work and/or chemotherapy. During the waiting period it is thus not known whether the patient will require further treatment, although most patients would expect to undergo venipuncture.

EMLA anesthesia could easily be introduced into this routine practice by applying the cream immediately after the capillary blood work. The waiting period that occurs before consultation with the physician, during analysis of capillary blood, would then coincide with the application time required for EMLA cream. Application of the cream at the hematology/oncology clinic would ensure that the cream is applied by the nurse ultimately responsible for carrying out the venipuncture. This is important in children with poor venous access, in whom locating a suitable site may be difficult. As the efficacy of EMLA cream increases with increasing application time, and only minor local effects are associated with its use, the potential for an application/waiting time longer than 60 minutes, or for cancelation of treatment requiring venipuncture, does not present a problem.

B. Neurology Clinic

Data from the neurology clinic reveal a mean patient waiting time of 60.2 ± 45.5 minutes (range 5 to 200 minutes), from the time children registered with the staff nurse to the time of venipuncture at the phlebotomy clinic. Nineteen of the 31 patients (61%) received their venipuncture prior to 61 minutes. From this group of nineteen, 11 of the patients received blood analysis between 45 and 60 minutes after registration with the neurology nurse, while the other 8 (25%) patients waited less than 45 minutes.

In many hospitals, neurology patients with prearranged blood analysis wait to be seen first by the clinic nurse and later by the consulting physician. Seventy-five percent of the patients reporting to the clinic studied by Robieux et al. [1] received venipuncture after a wait of 45 minutes or longer; EMLA cream could therefore be used in these patients with little or no change to the routine practice. The remaining 25% of patients, who wait less than 45 minutes, could be given the option of EMLA cream application if they deem the additional waiting time worth the reduction of pain during venipuncture.

C. Phlebotomy Station

The time interval between arrival at the phlebotomy station and venipuncture for children from the nephrology, gastroenterology, cardiology and rheumatology clinics ranged from 5 to 12 minutes, which is clearly less than the 60 minutes required for effective EMLA analgesia [1].

The use of EMLA cream would thus be feasible only with some modifications to the current routine of these clinics. Alternatively, EMLA cream could be applied at home, prior to attendance at the clinic.

III. EMLA APPLICATION AT HOME

The main advantage of home application of EMLA cream is the avoidance of any delay at the clinic incurred by the necessary 60-minute application time. However, there are several factors that must be taken into consideration before allowing EMLA cream to be used by unskilled individuals. Potential problems include the difficulty in choosing a suitable site for venipuncture and the requirement for applying the cream correctly (the thickness of the layer of cream and good occlusion with dressing are both important). Other factors, such as the timing of application of the cream at home and the total dose administered, are not so critical. EMLA cream is effective over 1 to 3 hours after application, and painless needle insertion can be performed over a long period after removal of the cream, which accommodates variability in clinical routine. In addition, the safety margin for toxicity of EMLA cream is very wide and an overdose with the cream is unlikely. Moreover, with the introduction of the unit-dose package known as the EMLA patch, the feasibility of applying the local anesthetic at home further increases.

A. Clinical Studies

A recent study by Olofsson et al. [2] evaluated the ability of parents to follow written instructions and apply EMLA cream at home to pediatric patients. The 228 consecutive patients (aged 1 to 15 years) enrolled in the study were due for ENT outpatient surgery. Parents received preoperative information that included a prescription for EMLA cream and instructions on how it should be applied. Immediately after surgery, parents were asked to complete a questionnaire detailing any difficulty encountered in choosing the site(s) of EMLA application, why the cream was or was not used, and their opinion of the written instructions. The anesthesiology nurse gave details of time and site of

EMLA cream application, ease of venipuncture and whether the site chosen for cream application could be used for the puncture.

Of the 228 patients enrolled, 23 were excluded from evaluation owing to failure in registration or failure to receive the prescription and instructions. Nearly all the parents (97%) of the remaining 205 patients had read the information provided, and 180 (88%) of these patients received EMLA cream. The main reason given for using the cream was "pain-free venipuncture." Parents of 25 (12%) patients chose not to apply EMLA cream, giving such reasons as: could withstand the pain ($n = 8$), did not reach the pharmacy ($n = 4$), children did not want the cream ($n = 2$), parents did not believe in its use ($n = 2$), other reasons ($n = 9$).

Of those parents who used EMLA cream, 170 (94%) had looked for veins before applying the cream. Only 23 (13%) reported that they had been unsure where to apply the cream. The majority of parents ($n = 146$, 81%) had applied the cream at two or more sites, the most common being the back of the hand. No information was recorded on the ease of application and adhesion of the occlusive dressing. The anesthesiology nurses' reports showed that in 159 (88%) patients, venipuncture through anesthetized skin was possible. For the remaining 21 (12%) patients, venipuncture was impossible through anesthetized skin, but in nine of these no suitable veins were found at any site.

Olofsson et al. [2] conclude that home use of EMLA cream is feasible and increases the efficiency of outpatient ENT surgery by eliminating waiting periods and making the patients more cooperative. However, the authors stress the importance of detailed preoperative written instructions.

In another study, completed recently by Taddio et al. [3], EMLA cream was applied at home to infants (aged 3 to 4 months) who were due to receive a second DPT vaccination, in a placebo-control blinded protocol. Parents were instructed to apply the supplied cream (EMLA or placebo) 60 minutes before attending the clinic. Parental compliance approached 100% and in only few cases was the occlusive Tegaderm® applied ineffectively. The parents reported that application of the cream was easy, and that they would be prepared to use it again in the future if required.

IV. EMLA PATCH

The EMLA patch is a single-unit dose (1 g) of EMLA in a foam adhesive package. It simplifies and speeds up the application of EMLA, because applying a thick layer of cream and covering it with a separate adhesive dressing can be messy. It also allows control of the dose administered per application, thus preventing over- or underdosing. The patch should facilitate application of EMLA in the home, and may allow nonprescription use of EMLA in a greater number of countries than is permitted at present.

A. Clinical Studies

To date, clinical trials with the EMLA patch have all involved hospital rather than home application. A number of trials have been reported that assess the efficacy, ease of application and adverse effects associated with the EMLA patch compared with EMLA cream plus Tegaderm dressing. Results from these studies, which are detailed below, indicate that the EMLA patch and cream formulations are similar in analgesic efficacy and rate of adverse reactions. Although some studies suggest that the EMLA patch does not adhere to the skin as effectively as Tegaderm dressing, this does not appear to affect efficacy.

Study 1

Robieux et al. [4] conducted a randomized, open-label comparison of the EMLA patch and EMLA cream in 160 children (aged 5 to 18 years) from four clinics at The Hospital for Sick Children in Toronto. The cream (2.5 g) was applied under an adhesive, occlusive tape (Tegaderm), and the patch was a standard package composed of EMLA (1 g) enclosed with foam tape adhesive. At the time of puncture, adhesiveness of the tape and local reactions were recorded. Pain experienced during removal of the tape and during venipuncture was scored by the patient on a visual analog scale (VAS) of zero (no pain) to 100 (worst imaginable pain).

Results from this study are reported in Table 1. The mean VAS for pain experienced during removal of the Tegaderm dressing was

Table 1 Comparison of EMLA Patch and EMLA Cream

	EMLA patch	EMLA cream plus Tegaderm
Number of patients	80	80
VAS for removal of dressing	19 ± 26	19 ± 21
VAS for venipuncture	8.5 ± 16	9.5 ± 17
No. of patients in whom tape was incompletely affixed at the end of application time	14 (18%)	5 (6%)

VAS = Visual analog scale.
Source: Ref 4.

very similar to that for removal of the EMLA patch. Likewise, there was no statistical difference in the VAS for venipuncture between the two groups. It is interesting to note that the amount of pain reported by the children following venipuncture was statistically less ($p <$ 0.001) than the pain experienced on removal of the adhesive tape. The frequency of local reactions was not statistically different between the two groups. The most common reactions were pallor at the site of the EMLA application and redness at the site of the adhesive tape, both of which were mild and transient. In two cases (one from each group) a more severe reaction occurred, which included an itchy rash lasting 2 days at the site of application.

At the time of removal of the dressing, the EMLA patch was incompletely attached to the skin in a greater number of cases than was the Tegaderm dressing over the cream. This was thought to be related to the stiffness of the foam tape of the EMLA patch, which could become loosened when applied close to a joint such as on the cubital fossa. The Tegaderm dressing was softer and more flexible, and thus more compatible with normal arm movement.

Study 2

A clinical trial recently reported by Nilsson et al. [5] compared the analgesic efficacy, adhesiveness and local skin reactions associated with the use of the EMLA patch and cream (2.5 g) plus Tegaderm dressing. The randomized, open, parallel-group study enrolled 63 children (aged 5 to 15 years), most of whom were due to undergo venipuncture for induction of anesthesia and who therefore received premedication during the EMLA application time. Three of the patients were later withdrawn from the study. Pain experienced during venipuncture was assessed by the patient using a 100 mm VAS. The investigators assessed both pain during venipuncture and discomfort during removal of the dressing using a 3-point verbal rating scale (VRS) of no pain, slight or severe pain. Local skin reactions caused by the dressing and EMLA were also noted.

Statistical analysis (analysis of variance) of the VAS scores reported by the patients indicated that the pain experienced by the patch and the cream groups could be regarded as equivalent, even though the median application time in the two groups differed (120 and 109 minutes, respectively). The verbal rating scores reported by the investigators also revealed no difference in the pain experienced on venipuncture between the patch and the cream groups; a score of "no pain" was given for 22 and 23 patients, respectively. Removal of the dressing was scored as "no pain" in 26 and 28 patients, respectively.

In this study [5], no difference was detected between the two groups with respect to the adhesiveness of the EMLA patch and Tegaderm; the dressing was intact in about 70% of patients in both groups. Local reactions to the dressing or EMLA anesthetic were also similar in both groups.

Study 3

Goresky and Klassen [6] recently reported the results from a cross-over study comparing EMLA cream (2.5 g) plus Tegaderm dressing with the EMLA patch (1 g standard dose) in 31 children undergoing phlebotomy and autologous transfusion. EMLA cream or patch was applied during one visit and the alternate treatment applied on the next visit; application times were 60 to 180 minutes. The adhesiveness of the dressing, discomfort on removal of the dressing, local skin reactions and pain during venipuncture were all assessed.

No significant differences were found between the two treatment arms for any of the parameters studied. Redness was common at the site of the dressing adhesive in both groups, as was pallor and redness at the EMLA contact site. Pain scores, rated by the patient and an observer, were similar in both groups. The dressing became partially separated from the skin in three patients receiving cream plus Tegaderm and in five patients from the EMLA patch arm of the trial. The large size of the EMLA patch resulted in some difficulty in maintaining full skin contact in younger patients.

Study 4

Similar results were seen in a multicenter trial involving 178 children, aged 3 to 10 years, reported by Chang et al. [7]. The nonpremedicated patients were randomized to receive either the patch (containing 1 g EMLA) or the cream (2.5 g) with Tegaderm dressing. Pain during removal of the dressing and during venipuncture was asessed using a 3-point VRS by both the patient and an observer. Assessments were also made for the adhesiveness of the dressing (5-point scale) and local reactions (4-point scale).

The patch and cream were equally effective in alleviating pain during venipuncture, with 95% and 94% of patients, respectively, reporting no or slight pain. There was also no statistical difference in the patients' rating of pain on removal of the dressing. The patch was found to be significantly less adhesive ($p = 0.001$) than the cream plus dressing, although this clearly had no effect on the efficacy of the patch. Local reactions included pallor and itching; there was no significant difference between the two groups.

V. DISCUSSION

The study of Robieux et al.[1] demonstrates that, in the hematology/ oncology clinic, EMLA cream can be effectively used for outpatients without changing routine practices or wasting time. In addition, relatively minor modifications in the routine of the neurology clinic can allow neurology patients to benefit from EMLA cream. However, regular use of the cream would not be feasible in nephrology, cardiology, rheumatology and gastroenterology clinics without some changes in current clinical practices. These results, coupled with numerous recent studies showing the efficacy of EMLA in providing analgesia during painful procedures, indicate that EMLA cream could benefit many pediatric outpatients without affecting routine clinical practices.

The waiting period required with the use of EMLA cream can be utilized to reduce the anxiety and fear caused by children's anticipation of painful procedures. For example, an anxious child can be told that some "magic cream" is going to be applied that will help to take the pain away [8]. Techniques such as distraction, visual imagery, and hypnotic suggestions that make the child envision the numbing action of the anesthetic, along with maternal affection, are also useful tools in attempts to lower the distress experienced by these children.

The EMLA patch is a single-dose, easy-to-apply product that yields a degree of analgesia similar to that of EMLA cream covered with Tegaderm. This mode may be especially useful for parents who wish to apply EMLA at home before bringing their child for a painful procedure such as venipuncture, as very limited patient or parental instruction is required. It is likely that, once in widespread use, the unit-dose package will prevent under- or overmedication in some cases. At present, use of the EMLA patch has been reported only during venipuncture, more studies are needed to test the effectiveness of this product in other procedures.

VI. CONCLUSION

While the hesitation to add EMLA to the routine practice of outpatient clinics is understandable, the data indicate that in most cases these doubts are not justified. It is our view that EMLA should be offered to every child experiencing repeated procedure-related pain and to selected groups of adults who wish to decrease the level of pain associated with such procedures.

REFERENCES

1. Robieux I, Kumar R, Radhakrishnan S, Koren G: The feasibility of using EMLA cream to relieve pain in pediatric outpatient clinics. Can J Hosp Pharm 1990; 43: 235-236.

2. Olofsson J, Guttormsen AB, Nordahl SHG: Improved efficacy of pediatric ENT outpatient surgery using home application of EMLA cream. Presented at the World ENT Congress, June 1993.
3. Taddio A, Nulman I, Goldoch M, et al.: Use of lidocaine-milocaine cream for vaccinations in infants. J Pediatr 1994; 124: 643-648.
4. Robieux I, Eliopoulos C, Hwang P, Greenberg M, Blanchette V, Olivieri N, Koren G: Pain perception and effectiveness of the eutectic mixture of local anesthetics in children undergoing venipuncture. Pediatr Res 1992; 32: 520-523.
5. Nilsson A, Engberg G, Rotstein A: A clinical study on a single unit dose package of EMLA (EMLA patch) and EMLA 5% cream used to reduce pain from venipuncture in children. Anaesthesia 1994; 49: 70-72.
6. Goresky GV, Klassen K: EMLA patch for phlebotomy in children. Anesth Analg 1993; 76: S121.
7. Chang PC, Goresky G, O'Connor GV, Pyesmany DA, Rogers PCJ, Stewart DJ, Stewart JA: A multicenter randomized study of single-unit dose package of EMLA patch vs. EMLA 5% cream used to reduce pain from venipuncture in children. Presented at the Annual Meeting of the Royal College of Physicians and Surgeons of Canada, September 1991.
8. MacKinlay GA: Save the prepuce. Painless separation of preputial adhesions in the outpatient clinic. Br Med J 1988; 297: 500-501.

6

EMLA for Neonatal Circumcision

Madlen Gazarian
The Hospital for Sick Children
Toronto, Ontario, Canada

I. INTRODUCTION

The practice of routine, nonreligious neonatal circumcision remains a controversial issue [1,2]. While attitudes have been shifting in the last 15 to 20 years, recent evidence tends to support the medical benefits of the procedure, particularly in the prevention of urinary tract infections (UTIs) in infant boys and sexually transmitted diseases (STDs) in young men [3]. However, medical considerations seem to play only a small role in the parental decision regarding circumcision [4–6], and the fact remains that in some countries up to 85% of boys are being circumcised [7–9]. The issue of pain during circumcision has itself been a target for controversy, and the majority of neonatal circumcisions continue to be performed without any form of anesthesia.

There is now ample evidence not only that the neonate is capable of experiencing pain but also that failure to provide adequate relief may in fact have adverse effects [10]. Thus, a safe, effective, painless and easy-to-use method of anesthesia for newborn circumcision would be most welcome by all concerned.

II. NEONATAL CIRCUMCISION: ONGOING CONTROVERSY

Circumcision is one of the oldest known surgical procedures and continues to be practiced by an estimated 25% of the world's population, including Jews and Moslems, black Africans, and Oceanians as well as Caucasians in North America and Europe [7]. Among the developed nations, the highest rate of circumcision is found in the United States, where it averages 85%. The lowest rate occurs in Scandinavian countries, where only 0.02% of boys are circumcised [11]. Canada and Australia have intermediate rates of about 45% [7]. These rates have been fluctuating in recent times [9]. An evaluation of the factors influencing the circumcision decision leads one to examine the attitudes of both the medical profession and parents toward the practice.

In the past, medical arguments for neonatal circumcision have centered on the possibility that the procedure may help to prevent certain diseases such as balanoposthitis, phimosis, carcinoma of the penis, carcinoma of the cervix and sexually transmitted diseases, including the heterosexual transmission of HIV as well as group B streptococcus [3,12]. The issue that has received most attention in recent times, however, is the strong association that has been found between the uncircumcised state and the occurrence of urinary tract infections in boys during the first 12 months of life [13]. A recent meta-analysis of nine studies evaluating the frequency of UTIs among boys less than 12 months of age revealed a statistically significant increase in the incidence of UTIs in the uncircumcised group. The odds ratios ranged from a five- to 89-fold increased risk for UTI in uncircumcised boys [14]. Some argue, however, that adequate penile hygiene could confer as much protection as neonatal circumcision

[1,2,15], although there seem to be no published studies to support this hypothesis [16].

The possible complications of neonatal circumcision include meatal stenosis, infection, hemorrhage and cosmetic disfigurement. There are many other potential problems [7,12], but these are quite rare in practice. In fact, the reported complication rate is quite low, ranging between 0.2 and 0.6% [17], with the most common being local infection and bleeding. Pain and possible psychological trauma associated with the procedure are also important factors in the argument against the practice of neonatal circumcision.

In the light of the emerging data regarding UTIs, the American Academy of Pediatrics (AAP) recently revised its stand on the circumcision of newborns. The report of the Task Force [17] concludes by stating: "Newborn circumcision has potential medical benefits and advantages as well as disadvantages and risks. When circumcision is being considered, the benefits and risks should be explained to the parents and informed consent obtained."

The impact that prevailing medical attitudes toward circumcision has on parents is difficult to estimate. Brown and Brown [4] tested the hypothesis that parents based their circumcision decision predominantly on social rather than medical concerns. They surveyed parents of 124 newborns soon after they made the circumcision decision to learn their reasons for the decision. The strongest factor associated with the circumcision decision was whether the father was circumcised. The research also showed that parents' concerns about the attitudes of peers and their sons' self-concept in the future were prominent in the decision to circumcise. Similar findings are reported by King et al. [6], in whose study concerns regarding hygiene and the need to conform with the father or male siblings figured highly. In contrast, only 4% of mothers gave possible medical advantage as a reason for wanting circumcision.

While a definitive judgment is awaited on the medical indication for routine neonatal circumcision, parents will continue to be influenced by religious, cultural and traditional factors. Hence, as Stang et al. [18] contend, "If, despite parent education, circumcisions are still to be performed, we owe it to our children to perform them as humanely as possible." Alternatively, one could argue that the recent change in the AAP stand on newborn circumcision may prompt a resurgence in the popularity of the procedure, making the question of pain relief even more relevant to a larger group of individuals [19].

III. PAIN IN CIRCUMCISION

Newborn circumcision has been performed without any form of anesthesia through the centuries and remains the "standard" practice to this day. The justification for this approach lay in the traditional view that the neonate was not capable of experiencing pain. However, this is now known not to be the case ([10]; see also Chapter 3). The physiological markers associated with pain or nociceptive activity in the neonate include changes in heart rate, blood pressure [20], metabolism and hormone levels [10], decreased oxygenation [21] and increased palmar sweating [22]. Behavioral responses of neonates toward pain include distinct facial expressions and cry patterns, and alterations in more complex behavior and sleep-wake cycles [23–26] (see Chapter 3).

A. Studies of Pain During Circumcision

In neonates circumcised without anesthesia, cortisol levels have been shown to rise markedly during and after the procedure [27,28], and in neonates undergoing circumcision, the use of local anesthesia has been found to be effective in reducing the physiological markers of stress [20] as well as in modifying the adrenocortical stress response [18].

Marshall et al. [29] evaluated the effect of circumcision on the behavior of 26 infants in a double-blind, randomized, controlled study using the Brazelton Neonatal Behavior Assessment Scale. They found that nearly 90% of the circumcised infants had altered behavioral states following the procedure, compared to only 16% of the control group. One-third of those with altered behavior continued to demonstrate these changes up to 22 hours after circumcision. In a subsequent study it was shown that there were also alterations in the mother-infant interaction immediately following circumcision [30]. These included differences in feeding patterns as well as in the availability of the infants for social interaction. While the measured differences in this group had resolved by 24 hours postoperatively, another study found that behavioral differences were still evident on the day following the procedure [31]. The latter study also showed that infants receiving local anesthesia in the form of a dorsal penile nerve block remained more attentive following circumcision and demonstrated a greater ability to quiet themselves when disturbed.

It is interesting to speculate on the possible longer-term effects of newborn circumcision without anesthesia [32]. Some contend that since newborns have a much greater capacity for memory than was previously thought, painful experiences in the neonatal period could possibly lead to psychological sequelae in the long term [10,33,34].

B. Use of Analgesia

Despite the evidence that neonates perceive pain and that the outcome of painful procedures is better when analgesia is employed, the vast majority of physicians performing newborn circumcision either do not employ analgesics or use agents of questionable efficacy [35]. A recent survey of 171 family physicians and pediatricians revealed that, of the 40% who performed newborn circumcisions, only a minority (24%) used any form of analgesia. The most common agent (20%) was ethanol, given as a small dose of whiskey. The remaining 4% of physicians used dorsal penile nerve block; no other form of analgesia was used. The most common reasons given for not using analgesia were lack of familiarity with analgesics used in neonates (59%), lack of familiarity with the technique of dorsal penile nerve block (53%) and concern over the adverse effects of analgesics (50%). Interestingly, the procedure was not felt to warrant the use of analgesia by 47% of those performing circumcisions, while 40% felt that neonates had a reduced experience of pain compared to older children and adults [35]. Thus, it seems that misconceptions about the neonatal experience of pain are still prevalent within the medical profession.

The accumulating body of evidence leads one to conclude that the newborn is capable of experiencing nociception, and antinociceptive measures improve clinical outcome following neonatal surgery. It is also clear that the pain experience itself cannot be measured in the newborn; the degree of suffering can only be estimated by observers. However, as indicated by Boreus [34], there remain at least two fundamental reasons to give analgesia in the newborn: 1) humanitarian —to alleviate assumed suffering and 2) medical—to improve the result of treatment.

IV. ANESTHETIC AGENTS FOR NEONATAL CIRCUMCISION

The consideration of anesthesia for circumcision in the neonatal period leads inevitably to an evaluation of the risk:benefit ratio of the agent in question. Due to the functional immaturity of the respiratory, cardiovascular and central nervous systems, there is an increased risk from narcotic and general anesthesia for newborn infants [19]. The anesthetic mortality rate for newborns may be as high as 1 in 1000 [36]. Thus, while general anesthesia would be the most effective method of relieving pain, the associated risks are clearly unacceptable for newborn circumcision. Safer alternatives are available but as yet none has gained wide acceptance.

A. Dorsal Penile Nerve Block (DPNB)

The DPNB as a technique for local anesthesia during routine neonatal circumcision was first introduced by Kirya and Werthmann in 1978 [37]. It involves subcutaneous injection of a total of 0.4 to 0.8 ml of lidocaine solution (1%) at two sites over the dorsal nerves near the penile root. Subsequent evaluations of the technique have shown that it is effective in reducing physiological and behavioral signs of distress both during and following circumcision [18,20,31]. However, the technique is not widely utilized [35].

One reason given by physicians for not using the DPNB is that the pain or stress of the injection itself may offset the beneficial effects of the local anesthesia. This was not found to be the case in a study by Stang et al. [18], who evaluated the behavioral and adrenocortical responses of 60 neonates undergoing circumcision with DNPB ($n = 20$), normal saline injection ($n = 20$) or no injection ($n = 20$). The authors found that injection of fluid during the procedure did not by itself increase the pain and stress experienced by the neonate.

Another reason cited for concern regarding the DPNB is that it may add risks to an already elective procedure. Possible complications may include hematomas, gangrene of the surface of the glans, localized bleeding at the puncture sites and transient vasoconstriction and ischemia of the genitalia [19,38–40]. Inadvertent injection of lidocaine into the dorsal penile vein or one of the arteries, as well as possible systemic toxicity following absorption of lidocaine injected into the tissues, are also theoretical problems [19]. While the latter complication has not yet been reported, the possibility of its occurrence remains a cause for concern [16]. Thus, Schoen and Fischell [19] advocate caution in the use of this technique until large studies demonstrating its safety have been performed.

B. Topical Anesthesia

Lidocaine

Weatherstone et al. [41] recently evaluated the use of 30% lidocaine cream as a topical anesthetic for routine circumcision in healthy, full-term newborns. The anesthetic cream was applied for 20 minutes in 12 babies. The control group (eight babies) received an acid mantle cream placebo. The variables that were studied included: vital signs such as respiratory rate, heart rate, blood pressure and oxygen saturation; behavioral changes; and serum β-endorphin levels. There was no difference in vital signs between the treatment and control groups throughout the study period. However, the treatment group had significantly fewer behavioral and serum β-endorphin level changes when compared to the control group. There was minimal systemic absorption of lidocaine, and no adverse side effects were reported. While these results are encouraging, the numbers studied are too small from which to draw firm conclusions.

EMLA

EMLA$^{®}$ cream has been used successfully for the painless separation of preputial adhesions in older boys (aged 2 to 12 years) who would otherwise have required circumcision. MacKinlay [42] studied a group of 39 boys referred for circumcision, none of whom had a retractable foreskin. EMLA cream was applied under an occlusive dressing for 60 minutes; then the adhesions were separated with a probe and gauze swab. The procedure was completely pain-free in 32 boys, seven had mild discomfort and only one boy shed tears. One boy required a repeat procedure and another had to undergo circumcision later because of fibrous phimosis. No signs of toxicity were encountered, although plasma concentrations of lidocaine and prilocaine were not measured.

More recently, Benini et al. [43] evaluated the efficacy of EMLA cream as an anesthetic agent in 27 newborns undergoing circumcision. The babies were randomly assigned to receive EMLA (0.5 g, not 0.05 g as reported in Ref. 43 [C. C. Johnston, personal communication] or placebo cream 45 to 60 minutes prior to the circumcision. Heart rate, transcutaneous oxygen saturation, facial activity and cry power spectra were continuously recorded throughout the procedure. Compared to baseline, all babies experienced pain during all phases of the procedure, as evidenced by increased heart rate, decreased oxygen saturation and more facial actions indicative of pain. When compared to placebo, EMLA cream was found to significantly attenuate the pain response, as indicated by lower heart rate and higher oxygen saturation, particularly during the clamping and lysis phases. However, there was no significant difference in heart rate or oxygen saturation between groups during cutting of the foreskin. Interpretation of the facial action scores and percentage of time spent crying during the procedure was difficult because the groups had different baseline values, with the placebo group having a higher facial action score and crying more than the EMLA group even before the procedure started. The cry power spectra showed no differences between the two groups. Once again, the numbers studied were small; it is therefore difficult to draw firm conclusions.

No untoward clinical effects from EMLA cream were noted; however, any changes in methemoglobin levels were not reported in this study. As detailed in Chapter 2, newborn infants have a higher susceptibility to methemoglobinemia due to the immaturity of the methemoglobin reductase system at this age. Thus, the safety of EMLA cream, especially in relation to methemoglobin production, will have to be studied before it can be recommended for use as a local anesthetic in newborn infants. (At present the internationally recommended age limit for use of EMLA is 3 months, although some countries have adopted higher or lower limits.) Several large-scale clinical trials are planned to start in the near future, designed to study the efficacy and safety of EMLA cream in neonatal circumcision.

Safety concerns have also been addressed by Gazarian et al. [unpublished observations] in an in vivo study to evaluate EMLA cream using a piglet model. The piglet was chosen because of its metabolic similarities to humans in the handling of local anesthetics and other drugs. The extent of drug absorption and consequent o-toluidine and methemoglobin formation was measured after a 1 hour application of EMLA cream (1 g) to the penile skin of 15 newborn piglets. Values were compared to those achieved after equivalent doses of lidocaine and prilocaine (25 mg of each) were administered intravenously. Following penile application of EMLA cream, the mean bioavailabilities of prilocaine and lidocaine were 9.6% and 4.0%, respectively. The amount of o-toluidine produced after intravenous administration of prilocaine was nearly 60-fold greater than that produced after topical application of EMLA cream. The mean maximum methemoglobin value after i.v. administration was 1.23 ± 0.64%, compared to 0.99 ± 0.36% after topical penile application. The elevation in methemoglobin above baseline was statistically significant after the i.v. doses of lidocaine and prilocaine and after penile application of EMLA cream ($p = 0.03$). However, in no cases did the elevation reach clinical significance. These findings suggest that the margin of safety with the use of EMLA cream at this dosage is quite wide, and it is hoped that similar safety data will be demonstrated in the forthcoming trials in human neonates.

C. Other Measures

Other potential forms of anesthesia for circumcision include acetaminophen, cryoanalgesia [19] and local infiltration of the foreskin with lidocaine [16,44]. Blass and Hoffmeyer [45] showed that the use of sucrose on a pacifier prior to and during circumcision reduced the amount of crying. Gunnar et al. [46] found that stimulating the newborn with a pacifier alone during circumcision also reduced crying, but there was no significant effect on the adrenocortical response. The absence of crying does not necessarily imply the absence of pain, and non-nutritive sucking may, at best, be viewed as a useful adjunct in relieving the distress of circumcision. Another intervention that should be considered is a reduction in the amount of restraint during the procedure, which itself adds to the total distress of the experience [43].

V. CONCLUSION

In conclusion, there is now little doubt that circumcision inflicts severe pain on the newborn infant and that a safe and effective form of anesthesia should be sought for use in this age group. The only published report on the use of EMLA during newborn circumcision suggests that the cream alleviates some of the pain associated with the procedure. More widespread use of EMLA cream for this indication must await safety studies in the human neonate followed by more confirmatory studies of efficacy.

REFERENCES

1. Wiswell TE, Metcalf T: Challenging opinions: Do you favor routine neonatal circumcision? Postgrad Med 1988; 84: 98-108.
2. Poland RL: The question of routine neonatal circumcision. N Engl J Med 1990; 322: 1312-1315.
3. Schoen EJ: The status of circumcision of newborns. N Engl J Med 1990; 322: 1308-1312.
4. Brown MS, Brown CA: Circumcision decision: Prominence of social concerns. Pediatrics 1987; 80: 215-219.
5. Coran AG: Circumcision in the United States: medical and nonmedical attitudes. Pediatr Surg Int 1989; 4: 229-230.
6. King PA, Caddy GM, Cohen SH, Pacca LE: Circumcision: Maternal attitudes. Paediatr Surg Int 1989; 4: 222-226.
7. Poenaru D: The circumcision controversy: A review. Univ Toronto Med J 1985; 62: 32-36.
8. Scharli AF: Circumcision, an everlasting discussion. Pediatr Surg Int 1989; 4: 221.
9. Wiswell TE, Hachey WE: Urinary tract infections (UTIs) and the uncircumcised state: an update (abstract 604). Pediatr Res 1992; 31: 103A.

10. Anand KJS, Hickey PR: Pain and its effects in the human neonate and fetus. N Engl J Med 1987; 317: 1321-1329.

11. Wallerstein E: In: Circumcision: An American health fallacy. Springer, New York, 1980.

12. Robson WLM, Leung AKC: The circumcision question. Postgrad Med 1992; 91: 237-244.

13. Wiswell TE, Roscelli JDR: Corroborative evidence for the decreased incidence of urinary tract infections in circumcised male infants. Pediatrics 1986; 78: 96-99.

14. Wiswell TE, Hachey WE: Urinary tract infections (UTIs) and the uncircumcised state: a meta-analysis (abstract 603). Pediatr Res 1992; 31: 103A.

15. Committee on Fetus and Newborn: Report of the Ad Hoc Task Force on Circumcision. Pediatrics 1975; 56: 610-611.

16. Wiswell TE: Circumcision: An Update. Curr Prob Pediat 1992; 22: 424-431.

17. AAP Task Force on Circumcision Report of the Task Force on circumcision. Pediatrics 1989; 84: 388-391.

18. Stang HJ, Gunnar MR, Snellman L, Condon LM, Kestenbaum R: Local anesthesia for neonatal circumcision. Effects on distress and cortisol response. J Am Med Assoc 1988; 259: 1507-1511.

19. Schoen EJ, Fischell AA: Pain in neonatal circumcision. Clin Pediatr 1991; 30: 429-432.

20. Williamson PS, Williamson ML: Physiological stress reduction by a local anesthetic during newborn circumcision. Pediatrics 1983; 71: 36-40.

21. Rawlings DJ, Miller PA, Engel RR: The effect of circumcision on transcutaneous pO_2 in term infants. Am J Dis Child 1980; 134: 676-678.

22. Harpin VA, Rutter N: Development of emotional sweating in the newborn infant. Arch Dis Child 1982; 57: 691-695.

23. Grunau RVE, Johnston CC, Craig KD: Neonatal facial and cry responses to invasive and non-invasive procedures. Pain 1990; 42: 295-305.

24. Emde RN, Harmon RJ, Metcalf D et al.: Stress and neonatal sleep. Psychosom Med 1971; 33: 491-497.

25. Porter FL, Miller RH, Marshall RE: Neonatal pain cries: Effect of circumcision on acoustic features and perceived urgency. Child Dev 1986; 57: 790-802.

26. Editorial. Pacifiers, passive behavior, and pain. Lancet 1992; 339: 275-276.

27. Talbert LM, Kraybill EN, Potter HD: Adrenal cortical response to circumcision in the neonate. Obstet Gynecol 1976; 48: 208-210.

28. Gunnar MR, Fisch RO, Korsvik S, Donhowe JM: The effects of circumcision on serum cortisol and behavior. Psychoneuroendocrinology 1981; 6: 269-275.

29. Marshall RE, Stratton WC, Moore JA, Boxerman SB: Circumcision. I: Effects upon newborn behavior. Infant Behav Dev 1980; 3: 1-14.

30. Marshall RE, Porter FL, Rogers AG, Moore JA, Anderson B, Boxerman SB: Circumcision. II: Effects upon mother-infant interaction. Early Human Dev 1982; 7: 367-374.

31. Dixon S, Snyder J, Holve R, Bromberger P: Behavioral effects of circumcision with and without anesthesia. J Dev Behav Pediatr 1984; 5: 246-250.

32. Richards MPM, Bernal J, Brackbill Y: Early behavior differences: Gender or Circumcision. Dev Psychobiol 1975; 9: 89-95.

33. Owens ME: Pain in infancy: conceptual and methodological issues. Pain 1984; 20: 213-230.

34. Boreus LO: Pain in the newborn: Pharmacodynamic aspects. Dev Pharmacol Ther 1990; 15: 142-148.

35. Wellington N, Rieder MI: Attitudes regarding analgesia for circumcision. Clin Invest Med 1991; 14: A21.

36. Gregory GA: Outcome of pediatric anesthesia. In: Pediatric Anesthesia. Gregory GA (ed). 2nd edn. New York: Churchill Livingstone, 1989; 1: 15-23.

37. Kirya C, Werthmann MW: Neonatal circumcision and penile dorsal nerve block: A painless procedure. J Pediatr 1978; 96: 998-1000.

38. Fontaine P, Toffler WL: Dorsal penile nerve block for newborn circumcision. Am Fam Physician 1991; 43: 1327-1333.

39. Sara CA, Lowry CJ: A complication of circumcision and dorsal nerve block of the penis. Anaesth Intensive Care 1984; 13: 79-85.

40. Berens R, Pontus SP: A complication associated with dorsal penile nerve block. Reg Anaesth 1990; 15; 309-310.

41. Weatherstone KB, Rasmussen LB, Erenberg A, Leff RD: Safety and efficacy of topical anesthesia for circumcision. Pediatr Res 1991; 29: 238A.

42. MacKinlay GA: Save the prepuce. Painless separation of preputial adhesions in the outpatient clinic. Br Med J 1988; 297: 590-591.

43. Benini F, Johnston CC, Faucher D, Aranda JV: Topical anesthesia during circumcision in newborn infants. J Am Med Assoc 1993; 270: 850-853.

44. Masciello AL: Anesthesia for neonatal circumcision: Local anesthesia is better than dorsal penile nerve block. Obstet Gynecol 1990; 75: 834-838.

45. Blass EM, Hoffmeyer MA: Sucrose as an analgesic for newborn infants. Pediatrics 1991; 87: 215-218.
46. Gunnar MR, Fisch RO, Malone S: The effects of a pacifying stimulus on behavioral and adrenocortical responses to circumcision in the newborn. J Amer Acad Child Psychol 1984; 23: 34-38.

7

Use of EMLA Cream as a Local Anesthetic for Laceration Repair

Michael J. Rieder

University of Western Ontario
London, Ontario, Canada

I. INTRODUCTION

The relief of pain and the therapy of painful conditions is one of the most common reasons for children to attend emergency departments [1], and it is a regrettable fact that the therapy of many conditions that present to emergency departments involves the potential for creating more pain [2,3], one of the most obvious examples being repair of lacerations with sutures.

On a seasonal basis, lacerations can account for as many as one-third of all injuries presenting to pediatric emergency departments. Although new developments in skin glues and tapes offer a potential for reducing the number of lacerations that require closure with sutures, many cases still require sutures to provide optimal cosmetic and functional results. A traditional practice of closing lacerations in children without anesthesia is mentioned only to be condemned, as it is now accepted that even young infants can experience pain and distress [4]. The current standard is to infiltrate the wound with a local anesthetic prior to laceration repair [5]. Amide anesthetics are generally employed for this indication, lidocaine being the one most commonly used in pediatric patients. Infiltration with local anesthetics provides rapid, effective anesthesia in the area of infiltration and, when performed with a moderate degree of care, is not associated with any toxic effects [5]. However, despite the safety and efficacy of this practice, it is not an ideal form of anesthesia for a number of reasons.

Infiltration of local anesthetic is performed using a needle, the sight of which can cause considerable anxiety and distress to children, particularly if the child has had previous unfortunate experiences with injections [6,7] (see Chapter 3). The use of a small-gauge needle may not be appreciated by children, because they often have an exaggerated view of a needle's size [8–10]. This fear can produce an atmosphere that increases the stress associated with laceration repair. The injection itself can be painful, especially if the solution is infiltrated rapidly into the tissues. The pH of unbuffered local anesthetics produces an unpleasant sensation in the tissues [4]. Although this can be relieved somewhat by increasing the pH of the local anesthetic, the stability of the solution can be affected, which is undesirable if a multi-dose container is used [11]. The child is often restrained during the procedure, which increases anxiety and distress. Children requiring restraint are often younger and less able to understand the rationale for wound closure; in addition, younger children may have a lower tolerance to pain than older children [6,12]. The infiltration of a local anesthetic under the wound can distort the wound edges, with the potential for difficulty in correct approximation of the wound edge. These problems can be exacerbated if the individual carrying out the infiltration and repair is relatively inexperienced in the care of children.

These considerations are important in the rational management of painful procedures in children. Distress and anxiety related to previous experiences is a major component of the perceived pain with future experiences. Many children describe the most unpleasant and painful part of laceration repair as the infiltration of the local anesthetic: hardly a desirable situation! This can have a negative effect on future experiences with a painful procedure or experience [1–4]. For these reasons, there has been considerable interest for some time in the development of topical local anesthetics for wound repair.

II. TOPICAL ANESTHETICS IN WOUND REPAIR

As discussed in Chapter 2, the development of effective topical local anesthetics has been problematic until recently [13–15]. The interest in topical anesthesia for laceration repair turned from the consideration of preparations with a single agent to combination formulations [1,4]. The more effective of these are described below.

A. TAC

A mixture of tetracaine, epinephrine (adrenaline) and cocaine, known by the acronym TAC, was studied in the late 1970s and early 1980s for use as a topical anesthetic during laceration repair [16–23]. This solution, which is not available commercially, must be prepared locally in the hospital pharmacy using readily available—but potentially very harmful—ingredients, including cocaine and epinephrine [2].

When used clinically, this solution is soaked into a gauze, which is then applied directly to the wound and held in place for several minutes (a dose of 3 to 5 ml is suggested for a 3 cm laceration [2]). The wound can then be probed to determine the extent and depth of local anesthesia. Gloves must be worn when handling TAC to avoid absorption of the components, most notably cocaine, by the individual administering the solution [2].

A number of studies have shown that TAC is effective in producing adequate analgesia in about 75 to 95% of the patients in whom it was used as a local anesthetic [16–23]. Its efficacy appears to be equivalent to that of lidocaine infiltration for facial wounds, but Hegenbarth et al. [22] demonstrated that for wounds in the extremities TAC is less effective than lidocaine infiltration (adequate analgesia was produced in 43 and 89% of patients, respectively).

In common with other preparations containing epinephrine, TAC cannot be used in extremities, and should be avoided in mucous membranes or near the eyes [2]. The very serious adverse effects of TAC, which include death, are related primarily to its absorption into the central circulation [23,24]. Following the use of TAC in normal clinical doses, the majority of patients have low but detectable levels of cocaine in the blood. The concentration of cocaine is sufficient to produce a positive urine screening test for 2 days after TAC administration. However, these concentrations have not been associated with changes in heart rate or blood pressure compared to controls [25–27]. In contrast, it is unusual to detect tetracaine in the blood of patients who have been treated with TAC in typical anesthetic doses [26,27].

Modifications of the TAC formula have been evaluated to determine whether a safer product can be developed. Dilution of the solution 50:50 with normal saline appears to confer equivalent anesthetic effects [28]. Removal of the tetracaine component does not appear to affect the efficacy of the solution significantly, while removal of the cocaine component significantly reduces anesthetic efficacy [29,30]. Preparations containing only cocaine also provide significantly less adequate anesthesia than does TAC [31]. An animal study has suggested that there may be a higher infection rate associated with TAC use, but this has not been supported by experience with humans [16–23,32].

Thus, TAC appears to be an effective topical anesthetic for laceration repair involving the face and scalp. Care must be taken on the part of the individual administering TAC to avoid transdermal absorption of TAC into the circulation. The use of TAC for lacerations on the face and scalp would be expected to be associated with systemic absorption of small amounts of cocaine, and on rare occasions may be associated with serious adverse events, including death. The fact that TAC must be prepared locally may make widespread use of this formulation difficult.

B. EMLA

EMLA$^{®}$ cream has been used for anesthesia in a number of procedures involving the skin, including venipuncture, lumbar puncture and reservoir access, as well as for curettage of molluscum contagiosum

[33–36]. The utility of this agent for these indications suggested that it might be useful as a topical anesthetic for laceration repair. EMLA cream has been demonstrated to be safe and effective when used as a topical anesthetic over intact skin, but there has been rather less experience with EMLA on broken skin. EMLA sterile cream should be used in all studies of anesthesia in wound repair.

The possible effects of EMLA cream on wound repair and the infectious complications of laceration repair have been investigated in a number of in vivo studies. The efficacy of EMLA for laceration repair in a clinical setting has been investigated by Nykanen et al. [38]; no other clinical studies of EMLA in this indication have been reported to date.

In Vivo Studies

Nykanen et al. [5] used a rat model to compare the effect of EMLA and lidocaine infiltration on wound healing. After general anesthesia was administered, controlled clean surgical lacerations were created and then closed in the presence of EMLA cream or lidocaine infiltration. No short-term toxicity was observed in either group, and there was no histological or clinical evidence of necrosis in any of the wounds when observed over a 14-day period. There was also no difference in the appearance of the scars produced in the two groups. The authors concluded that EMLA did not produce a detrimental effect on wound healing when used for the repair of clean wounds [5].

Powell et al. [37] noted that EMLA demonstrated antibacterial properties in vitro. However, when EMLA cream was added to wounds contaminated with a bacterial innoculum in a guinea pig model, Powell et al. found that the use of EMLA was associated with a wider zone of infection, a higher incidence of gross infection and a higher bacterial count compared to the use of a saline control (comparisons with other commonly used local anesthetics were not made in this study). For wounds that had not been infected, the wound breaking strength was greater in the EMLA-treated group than in controls. The authors did not specify whether sterile EMLA cream had been used during these investigations. These observed effects were attributed to an adverse effect of EMLA cream on host defenses. The results from this animal study suggest that EMLA cream should be used with caution, if at all, in infected wounds.

Clinical Study

Nykanen et al. [38] compared the efficacy of EMLA cream vs. placebo in providing topical anesthesia in a randomized, placebo-controlled, double-blind trial that permitted lidocaine supplementation where necessary. A total of 45 children (average age 9 years) presenting to the pediatric emergency department at the Children's Hospital of Western Ontario for repair of lacerations were enrolled. The lacerations were all fresh (within 12 hours of injury), and none of the patients had conditions associated with an increase in risk for wound infection, such as diabetes. EMLA cream or placebo was applied under an occlusive dressing for 40 minutes, after which the wound was probed to determine the depth of anesthesia and lidocaine infiltration given if necessary. The pain associated with laceration repair was assessed by the patients after the procedure using a visual analog scale (VAS) of 0 to 100.

The results from this study are summarized in Table 1. Lidocaine infiltration was required by a greater number of patients in the placebo group than in the EMLA group, although over half (66%) of the EMLA group required supplementary analgesia, primarily of the skin at the wound edge. In the wound itself, adequate analgesia was achieved in 81% of the patients given EMLA. There was no difference in the VAS score between the EMLA and placebo groups. A small number of patients in both groups had minor skin reactions, pallor being the most common. Wound infection was seen on follow-up in two patients, one from the placebo and one from the EMLA group [38].

This study demonstrated that there was no significant risk of adverse drug reactions and that the use of EMLA cream in clean, uncomplicated lacerations was not associated with an increased risk of wound infection. In the wound itself, the efficacy of a 40-minute application of EMLA cream was equivalent to that of TAC. However, there was insufficient analgesia in the intact skin bordering the wound edge in a number of the patients in the EMLA group, who then required supplemental lidocaine infiltration. Absorption of EMLA

Table 1 Comparison of EMLA Versus Placebo as a Topical Anesthetic for Laceration Repair

Characteristic	Placebo	EMLA
n	21	24
No. of patients requiring supplimental lidocaine infiltration	20	14
Post-procedure VAS for severity of pain	75 ± 51	86 ± 56
No. of patients with adverse events		
Pallor	3	7
Redness	1	2
Pruritis	1	2
Burning sensation	2	1

would be expected to be more rapid over the wound itself than through the adjacent intact skin. The efficacy of EMLA cream is dependent on the application time, with optimal anesthesia for intact skin being reached after 60 to 90 minutes [39]. In the above study, optimal analgesia may therefore not have been achieved.

It would be anticipated that an application time of 60 minutes would provide adequate analgesia of both the wound and the adjacent skin with no increase in risk for adverse reactions. Nykanen and co-workers are currently completing a double-blind, prospective, randomized clinical trial assessing the use of EMLA cream for laceration repair using this application time, and further research is in progress on the type of laceration for which EMLA would be most suitable.

III. DISCUSSION

The preliminary studies described above suggest that EMLA cream has great potential for anesthesia while undergoing laceration repair, and further studies are under way to expand the data on the use of EMLA for this indication. Adverse reactions associated with the use of EMLA for use in laceration repair are anticipated to be similar to those associated with its use for other indications, and are unlikely to be greater than those associated with conventional therapy. The results from one animal study suggest that EMLA cream may have a detrimental effect if applied to grossly contaminated or infected wounds, and for this reason it may be prudent to use EMLA cream only in clean wounds that are seen within 12 hours of when the injury was sustained.

Although the safety profile of EMLA cream appears to be much better than that of TAC, the experience with EMLA cream for use in laceration repair is too limited to provide a definitive answer as to which is preferable. TAC is less effective in providing anesthesia for wounds on the extremities than for those on the face or scalp, while preliminary studies suggest that EMLA cream is equally efficacious in peripheral and central sites. Studies comparing the efficacy and safety of TAC vs. EMLA cream for anesthesia during laceration repair will be necessary to resolve this issue. The fact that TAC must be prepared locally while EMLA is available commercially may make the use of EMLA easier for many facilities, especially if pharmacy resources are limited.

The time required for analgesia to take effect is an issue that, superficially, appears to be a major concern in an emergency department setting. However, this situation can be addressed by more innovative use of delays that are already present in the system. Many emergency departments have a triage station at which patients are initially assessed and then slotted in by priority for definitive treatment. Given that most lacerations are not life-threatening, it can be anticipated that there will be a waiting period for the vast majority of patients who present for laceration repair. Currently, the usual practice is that these patients and their parents sit and wait, which is a source of considerable frustration on the part of parents and a potential source of anxiety for patients. In a recent informal survey of Canadian pediatric emergency departments, we found that the average time a patient with lacerations waited after first presenting at triage until definitive repair was between 60 and 90 minutes. Clearly, this waiting time could be used constructively to provide analgesia for laceration repair. This would be advantageous for patients and physicians, and would be expected to be very popular with parents who are waiting for their child to be attended. If parents feel that this time is being used to provide anesthesia for their child that will avoid the need for a needle puncture, it is likely that their interactions with emergency department personnel will be more positive than they might have been otherwise! We are currently planning studies to address the efficacy and safety of routine use of EMLA cream for local anesthesia for laceration repair when given by nursing staff during triage.

IV. CONCLUSION

EMLA cream represents a new development that has important implications for the management of lacerations, a common problem for children presenting to emergency departments. Research is currently ongoing to define the optimal use of EMLA cream in laceration repair. Emergency departments that routinely treat children with lacerations should consider evaluating EMLA cream to determine if the use of this agent would be appropriate for their facility.

REFERENCES

1. Selbst SM, Henretig FM: The treatment of pain in the emergency department. Pediatr Clin North Am 1989; 36: 965-978.
2. Selbst SM: Managing pain in the pediatric emergency department. Pediatr Emerg Care 1989; 5: 56-63.
3. Berde CB: Pediatric post-operative pain management. Pediatr Clin North Am 1989; 36: 921-940.
4. Zeltzer LK, Anderson CTM, Schechter NL: Pediatric pain: current status and new directions. Curr Prob Pediatr 1990; 20: 411-486.
5. Nykanen D, Kissoon N, Rieder M, Armstrong R: Comparison of topical mixture of lidocaine and prilocaine (EMLA) versus 1% lidocaine inflitration on wound healing. Pediatr Emerg Care 1991; 7: 15-17.
6. Jay SM, Ozolins M, Elliot CH, Caldwell S: Assessment of children's distress during pain medical procedures. Health Psychol 1984; 2: 133-147.
7. Maher L, Mackie J: The incidence of post-operative pain in children. Pain 1983; 15: 271-282.
8. Lewis N: The needle is like an animal. Child Today 1978; 7: 18-21.
9. Menche E: School-aged children's perception of stress in the hospital. Child Health Care 1981; 9: 80-86.

10.   Fassler D, Wallace N: Children's fear of needles. Clin Pediatr 1982; 21: 59-60.

11.   Christoph RA, Buchanan L, Begallia K, Schwartz S: Pain reduction in local anesthetic administration through pH buffering. Ann Emerg Med 1988; 17: 117-120.

12.   Haslam DR: Age and the perception of pain. Psychonomic Sci 1969; 15: 86.

13.   Hille B: The common mode of action of three agents that decrease the transient change in sodium permeability in nerves. Nature 1966: 210: 1220-1222.

14.   Russo J, Lipman AG, Comslock TJ, Page BC, Stephen RL: Lidocaine anesthesia: comparision of iontophoresis, injection and swelling. Am J Hosp Pharm 1980; 37: 843-847.

15.   Lubens HM, Ausdenmoor RW, Schaffer AD, Reese RM: Anesthetic patch for painful procedures such as minor operations. Am J Dis Child 1974; 124: 192-194.

16.   Pryor GJ, Kilpatrick WR, Opp DR: Local anesthesia in minor lacerations: Topical TAC versus lidocaine infiltration. Ann Emerg Med 1980; 9: 568-571.

17.   Nichols FC, Macha P, Farnell MB: TAC topical anesthetic and minor skin lacerations. Resid Staff Phys 1987; 33: 59-66.

18.   Bonadio WA, Wagner V: Efficacy of TAC topical anesthesia for repair of pediatric lacerations. Am J Dis Child 1988; 142: 203-205.

19.   Bass DH, Wormald PJ, McNally J, Rode H: Topical anesthesia for repair of minor lacerations. Arch Dis Child 1990; 65: 1272-1273.

20.   Fitzmaurice LS, Wasserman GS, Knapp JF, Roberts DL, Waeckerle JF, Fox M: TAC use and absorption of cocaine in a pediatric emergency department. Ann Emerg Med 1990: 19: 515-518.

21.   Anderson AB, Colecchi C, Baronoski R, DeWitt TG: Local anesthesia in pediatric patients: topical TAC verus lidocaine. Ann Emerg Med 1990; 19: 519-522.

22.   Hegenbarth MA, Altieri MF, Hawk WH, Greene A, Ochsenschlager DW, O'Donnell R: Comparison of topical tetracaine, adrenaline and cocaine anesthesia with lidocaine inflitration for repair of lacerations in children. Ann Emerg Med 1990; 19: 63-67.

23.   Dronen SC: Complications of TAC. Ann Emerg Med 1983; 12: 333.

24.   Daily RH: Fatality secondary to misuse of TAC solution. Ann Emerg Med 1988; 17: 159-160.

25.   Altieri M, Bogema S, Schwartz RH: TAC topical anesthesia produces positive urine tests for cocaine. Ann Emerg Med 1990; 19: 577-579.

26. Terndrup TE, Mariani PJ, Walls HC, Spear RM, Karatay CM: Plasma cocaine and tetracaine levels following application of topical anesthesia in a swine laceration model. Am J Emerg Med 1991; 9: 539-543.

27. Terndrup TE, Walls HC, Mariani PJ, Gavula DP, Madden CM, Cantor RM: Plasma cocaine and tetracaine levels following application of topical anesthesia in children. Ann Emerg Med 1992; 21: 162-166.

28. Bonadio WA, Wagner V: Half strength TAC topical anesthetic. Clin Pediatr 1988; 27: 495-498.

29. Bonadio WA, Wagner V: Efficacy of tetracaine adrenaline cocaine topical anesthetic without tetracaine for facial laceration repair in children. Pediatrics 1990; 86: 856-857.

30. Schaffer DJ: Clinical comparison of TAC anesthetic solutions with and without cocaine. Ann Emerg Med 1985; 14: 1077-1080.

31. Ernst AA, Crabbe LH, Winsemius DK, Bragdon R, Link R: Comparison of tetracaine, adrenaline and cocaine with cocaine alone for topical anesthesia. Ann Emerg Med 1990; 19: 51-54.

32. Baker W, Rodenheaver GT, Edgertone MT, Edlich RF: Damage to tissue defences by a topical anesthetic agent. Ann Emerg Med 1982; 11: 307-310.

33. Hallen B, Carlsson P, Uppfelt A: Clinical study of lignocaine prilocaine cream to relieve the pain of venipuncture. Br J Anaesth 1985; 57: 326-328.

34. Manuksela EL, Korpella R: Double-blind evaluation of lignocaine prilocaine cream (EMLA) in children. Br J Anaesth 1986; 58: 1242-1245.

35. Rosdahl I, Edmar B, Gisslen H, Norden P, Lilliberg S: Curettage of molluscum contagiosum in children: analgesia by topical application of a lidocaine/prilocaine cream (EMLA). Acta Derm Venereol (Stockh) 1988; 68: 149-153

36. Halperin DL, Koren G, Attias D, Pellegrini E, Greenberg, Greenberg ML, Wyss M: Topical skin anesthesia for venous, subcutaneous drug reservoir and lumbar punctures in children. Pediatrics 1989; 2: 281-284.

37. Powell DM, Rodehaever GT, Foresman PA, Hankins CL, Belina KT, Zimmer CA, Becker DG, Edlich RF: Damage to tissue defences by EMLA cream. J Emerg Med 1991; 9: 205-209.

38. Nykanen D, Kissoon N, Rieder M, McGrath P: Efficacy of eutectic mixture of lidocaine and prilocaine (EMLA) as a topical anaesthetic agent in pediatric laceration repair. Ann Emerg Med. Submitted.

39. Juhlin L, Hagglund G, Evers H: Absorption of lidocaine and prilocaine after application of an eutectic mixture of local anaesthetics (EMLA) on normal and diseased skin. Acta Derm Venerol (Stockh) 1989; 69: 18-22.

8

Effect of Lidocaine-Prilocaine Cream (EMLA) on Injection and Vaccination Pain

Anna Taddio and Gideon Koren
The Hospital for Sick Children
Toronto, Ontario, Canada

I. INTRODUCTION

Although EMLA® cream has been investigated in many clinical indications [1–22] and has been extensively studied for use with venipuncture [1–9], little work has been reported to date on the potential
of EMLA cream for the alleviation of pain during vaccination. While
immunization programs for children of school age are well attended,
the percentage of infants who are vaccinated is low in some areas.

The poor uptake on vaccination programs for infants may be influenced by the pain associated with vaccination, which can, in the short term, affect the physical and mental well-being of children and their parents. The efficacy of EMLA cream in alleviating vaccination pain has therefore been assessed in a number of very recent studies, and this chapter presents the available data on the efficacy of EMLA cream in this indication.

In a preliminary investigation to determine whether EMLA cream would be suitable for use during vaccination, Taddio et al. carried out a clinical trial in adult volunteers that studied the pain experienced on needle prick and during subcutaneous (s.c.) injection of saline [23]. A second study was carried out in adults receiving an intramuscular (i.m.) injection of influenza virus vaccine [24]. At least two studies designed to assess the efficacy of EMLA cream in alleviating the pain of vaccination in infants have been carried out. These involved infants aged 3 to 28 months who were receiving diphtheria-pertussis-tetanus vaccines [25, 26]. A summary of the results from these studies is presented below.

II. SUBCUTANEOUS INJECTION

Taddio et al. [23] conducted a randomized, double-blind, cross-over study in 20 healthy adult volunteers. Each subject received both EMLA cream and a visually identical placebo cream (2.5 g under a Tegaderm® dressing), one cream on the left and one on the right arm, over the middle of the deltoid muscle. After an application time of 60 to 75 minutes, the dressings and creams were removed and local skin reactions, such as pallor, edema or redness, were rated by an investigator on a 4-point scale (absent, mild, moderate or severe). All injections were carried out by a single investigator; subjects received one s.c. injection of 0.9% sodium chloride (1.0 ml, room temperature) per site of cream application, administered with a 25-gauge needle at a 90° angle to the skin.

The pain associated with the needle puncture and the saline injection was scored by the subjects using separate ungraded visual analog scales (VAS) in which 0 mm denoted "no pain" and 100 mm denoted "worst possible pain." Needle puncture caused significantly less pain in the EMLA treated arms ($p < 0.01$); the median pain score for EMLA cream was 1 mm versus 4.5 mm for placebo. Injection pain was not statistically different between EMLA and placebo creams (median 7 mm and 4.5 mm, respectively), nor was it different between left and right arms. Needle puncture pain was statistically less than injection pain in EMLA-treated arms.

Twenty-two skin reactions were noted by the investigators in 17 (85%) of the EMLA-treated subjects; skin blanching occurred most frequently ($n = 13$). Seven (35%) of the placebo-treated subjects had eight skin reactions due to placebo cream; skin blanching was again the most frequent ($n = 3$).

III. INFLUENZA VIRUS VACCINATION

A randomized, double-blind trial was conducted by Taddio et al. [24] in 60 adults receiving Fluzone® influenza virus vaccine by i.m. injection. EMLA or placebo cream (2.5 g) was applied for 60 to 90 minutes, after which local skin reactions were rated using the 4-point scale described above. Subjects were then given Fluzone (0.5 ml, 2–8°C) using a 22-gauge needle inserted in the middle of the deltoid muscle at a 90° angle to the skin. (All injections were performed by two nurses familiar with the study protocol and blinded to treatment assignments.) The pain experienced during the needle prick and the injection were scored by the subjects using separate VAS.

The median pain scores in the EMLA group for both needle prick and injection were statistically lower than those reported by the placebo group (Table 1). The pain experienced during the needle prick was less than that experienced during vaccination in both the EMLA and the placebo groups, and there was a significant correlation between the two types of pain within each group. Significantly more subjects experienced local skin reactions in the EMLA group compared to placebo (97% vs. 48%, $p < 0.001$); however, these were mild and transient. Skin pallor was the most common reaction in the EMLA group and was observed in 21 subjects.

Table 1 Median Pain Scores for EMLA and Placebo Based on Visual Analog Scale (VAS) from 0 to 10 After Intramuscular Injection with Influenza Virus Vaccine

	EMLA ($n = 29$)	Placebo ($n = 31$)	p-value [a]
VAS (mm)			
Needle prick	1	8	< 0.0002
Injection	3	13	0.0139

[a] Mann-Whitney U test.

IV. VACCINATION PAIN IN INFANTS

A. Study 1

Taddio and co-workers have also carried out a randomized, double blind, placebo-controlled trial in infants receiving their 4-month or 6-month regular diphtheria-pertussis-tetanus (DPT®) vaccine [25]. EMLA or placebo cream (2.5 g) was applied to the vaccination site (i.e., upper thigh) by the infant's parent and covered by a Tegaderm® dressing for at least 60 minutes. Local skin reaction(s) were recorded on removal of the cream, then DPT vaccine (0.5 ml, 2–8 °C) was injected i.m. using a 25-gauge needle.

Each vaccination episode was videotaped for subsequent analysis of the degree of pain experienced. Pain was assessed by the investigators using two methods: a 100 mm unmarked VAS, scored within 15 seconds after the injection, and a modified behavioral pain scale (MBPS) [25]. The MBPS measures pain from three categories—the face, cry, and body movements; the total score varies from 0 to 10. Investigators measured the difference between the pre-injection (baseline) behavioral score, assessed within 5 seconds before injection, and the post-injection score, assessed up to 15 seconds afterward. Crying characteristics were assessed in terms of latency to first cry and total crying period.

Ninety-six infants (mean age 150 days; equal numbers of boys and girls) were evaluable for pain assessments; 49 were randomized

Table 2 Median Values for Infant Pain Scores and Crying Characteristics for EMLA and Placebo After Intramuscular Injection with Diphtheria-Pertussis-Tetanus Vaccine

	EMLA ($n = 49$)	Placebo ($n = 47$)	p-value [a]
Pre-vaccination MBPS score[b]	2	2	0.975
Post-vaccination MBPS score[b]	7	8	0.001
Difference (post- minus pre-vaccination MBPS score)	5	6	0.001
VAS pain score (mm)	26	48	0.002
Latency of first cry (seconds)	3.3	2.4	0.0004
Total length of cry (seconds)	10.3	25.2	0.027

[a] Mann-Whitney U test.
[b] Pain score assessed using a behavioral pain scale; see text.
Source: From Ref. 25.

to EMLA cream and 47 to placebo. Pain scores and crying characteristics are summarized in Table 2. The VAS score, the post-vaccination MBPS score and the difference between pre- and post-vaccination MBPS scores were all statistically lower for the EMLA group. EMLA subjects also had a longer latency to the first cry and a shorter total crying period compared to placebo. The difference in pre- and post-vaccination MBPS scores correlated with the VAS scores and with the total period of crying. It was noted that lower MBPS scores were associated with the girls in the study.

Adverse effects were evaluable for 50 subjects in the EMLA group and 49 in the placebo group. Ninety percent of EMLA-treated subjects experienced local skin reactions compared to 12% of placebo-treated subjects ($p < 0.0001$). Minor skin redness where the dressing had been applied occurred in 30% of the study sample. Skin blanching was the most common reaction with EMLA cream.

B. Study 2

A randomized, placebo-controlled, double-blind study carried out by Uhari [26] recruited 155 infants (mean age 9 months), most (98%) of

Table 3 Mean Values for Infant Pain Scores for EMLA and Placebo on Visual Scale from 0 to 10 Given by Nurses and Parents

	EMLA ($n = 79$)	Placebo ($n = 76$)	p-value [a]
Nurses' evaluation			
Pain	2.5	3.8	< 0.003
Crying	2.8	4.0	< 0.003
Parents' evaluation			
Pain	2.9	4.8	< 0.001
Crying	3.6	5.3	< 0.003

[a] Mann-Whitney U test.
Source: From Ref. 26.

whom were attending clinics for vaccination with diphtheria-pertussis-tetanus vaccine. EMLA or placebo cream was applied for a mean time of 65 minutes before vaccination. The amount of pain, crying and fear expressed by the infant was assessed by the parents and by the nurse administering the vaccine, using ungraded visual scales giving scores of 0 to 10. On returning home from the vaccination clinic, parents also assessed tenderness around the site of vaccination together with restlessness and elevated temperature.

The pain and crying scores for the EMLA-treated group, reported immediately after vaccination by both nurses and parents, were significantly lower than those for the placebo group (Table 3). As might be expected, there was no difference between the two groups in the score for fear. At home, parents reported significantly less tenderness at the site of vaccination in the EMLA-treated group, but there was no difference between the groups in the number of infants exhibiting restlessness or elevated temperature. In an overall assessment, the value of EMLA cream was rated higher than that of placebo cream, although there was an equal distribution between the two groups in the number of parents (71%) hoping that the cream would be used for the next vaccination. As reported in previous studies, skin paleness occurred more often in the EMLA group ($p < 0.01$).

V. CONCLUSION

When compared to placebo, EMLA cream decreased the pain elicited from the needle puncture in adults given either s.c. injections of normal saline or i.m. injections of Fluzone vaccine. EMLA cream also decreased the pain from infiltration of the Fluzone vaccine, but it did not decrease the pain from infiltration of the normal saline injection. These conflicting results can be explained by the differences in the characteristics of the two injected solutions, such as temperature, volume, pH, osmolality and method of administration. The observed correlation between needle and injection pain for the Fluzone vaccine suggests that the pain elicited by the needle may affect perception of the pain from the injection.

When compared to placebo in young infants receiving DPT vaccine, EMLA cream was associated with lower pain scores and a shorter duration of infant crying. EMLA cream therefore offers a new approach to the management of vaccination pain in infants. The consequences of these findings may extend well beyond the immediate post-vaccination period, as some investigators have suggested that painful events in young infants may have long-term consequences. Further research will be necessary to identify whether EMLA cream can prevent long-term adverse outcomes caused by painful procedures in infants.

Before general introduction of EMLA cream for the alleviation of vaccination pain, investigations should be carried out to assess the effect, if any, of EMLA on vaccine efficacy.

REFERENCES

1.   Hallen B, Uppfeldt A: Does lidocaine-prilocaine cream permit pain-free insertion of iv catheters in children? Anaesthesiology 1982; 57: 340-342.

2.	Halperin DL, Koren G, Attias D et al.: Topical skin anesthesia for venous, subcutaneous drug reservoir and lumbar punctures in children. Pediatrics 1989; 84: 281-284.

3.	Hopkins CS, Buckley CJ, Bush GH: Pain free injection in infants: use of lignocaine-prilocaine cream to prevent pain at intravenous induction of general anaesthesia in 1–5 year old children. Anaesthesia 1988; 43: 198-201.

4.	Manner T, Kanto J, Iisalo E et al.: Reduction of pain at venous cannulation in children with a eutectic mixture of lidocaine and prilocaine (EMLA® cream): comparison with placebo cream and no local premedication. Acta Anaesthesiol Scand 1987; 31: 735-739.

5.	Maunuksela EL, Korpela R: Double blind evaluation of a lignocaine-prilocaine cream (EMLA) in children: effect on the pain associated with venous cannulation. Br J Anaesth 1986; 58: 1242-1245.

6.	Wahlstedt C, Kollberg H, Moller C: Lignocaine-prilocaine cream reduces venepuncture pain. Lancet 1984; ii: 106.

7.	Kurien L, Kollberg H, Upperfeldt A: Venepuncture pain can be reduced. J Trop Med Hyg 1985; 88: 397-399.

8.	Soliman IE, Broadman LM, Hannallah RS et al.: Comparison of the analgestic effects of EMLA (eutectic mixture of local anesthetics) to intradermal lidocaine infiltration prior to venous cannulation in upremedicated children. Anaesthesiology 1988; 68: 804-806.

9.	Clarke S, Radford M: Topical anaesthesia for venepuncture. Arch Dis Child 1986; 61: 1132-1134.

10.	Juhlin L, Evers H, Broberg F: A lidocaine-prilocaine cream for superfical skin surgery and painful lesions. Acta Derm Venereol 1980; 60: 544-546.

11.	de Waard-van der Spek FB, Oranje AP, Lillieborg S et al.: Treatment of molluscum contagiosum using a lidocaine/prilocaine cream (EMLA) for analgesia. J Am Acad Dermatol 1990; 23: 685-688.

12.	Rosdhal I, Edmar B, Gisslen H et al.: Curettage of molluscum contagiosum in children: analgesia by topical application of a lidocaine prilocaine cream (EMLA®). Acta Derm Venereol 1988; 68: 149-153.

13.	Holm J, Andren B, Grafford K: Pain control in the surgical debridement of leg ulcers by the use of a topical lidocaine-prilocaine cream, EMLA®. Acta Derm Venereol 1990; 70: 132-136.

14.	Malmros IE, Nilsen T, Lillieborg S: Plasma concentrations and analgesic effect of EMLA® (lidocaine/prilocaine) cream for the cleansing of leg ulcers. Acta Derm Venereol 1990; 70: 227-230.

15. Lahteenmaki T, Lillieborg S, Ohlsen L et al.: Topical analgesia for the cutting of split-skin grafts: a multicenter comparison of two doses of a lidocaine/prilocaine cream. Plastic Reconstr Surg 1988; 82: 458-462.

16. Hallen A, Ljunghall K, Wallin J: Topical anaesthesia with local anaesthetic (lidocaine and prilocaine, EMLA) cream for cautery of genital warts. Genitourin Med 1987; 63: 316-319.

17. Ljunghall K, Lillieborg S: Local anaesthesia with a lidocaine/prilocaine cream (EMLA®) for cautery of condylomata acuminata on the vulval mucosa. The effect of timing of application of the cream. Acta Derm Venereol 1989; 69: 362-365.

18. Rylander E, Sjoberg I, Lillieborg S et al.: Local anesthesia of the genital mucosa with a lidocaine/prilocaine cream (EMLA) for laser treatment of condylomata acuminata: a placebo-controlled study. Obstet Gynecol 1990; 75: 302-306.

19. Sirimanna KS, Madden GJ, Miles S: Anaesthesia of the tympanic membrane: comparison of EMLA cream and iontophoresis. J Laryngol Otolaryngol 1990; 104: 195-196.

20. Roberts C, Carlin WV: A comparison of topical EMLA cream and prilocaine injection for anaesthesia of the tympanic membrane in adults. Acta Otolaryngol 1989; 108: 431-433.

21. Smith M, Gray BM, Ingram S et al.: Double blind comparison of topical lignocaine-prilocaine cream (EMLA) and lignocaine infiltration for arterial cannulation in adults. Br J Anaesth 1990; 65: 240-242.

22. Young AC, Shorthall A, Haynes W et al.: Lignocaine-prilocaine cream for lumbar puncture. Lancet 1987; ii: 1533.

23. Taddio A, Robieux I, Koren G: Effect of lidocaine-prilocaine cream on pain from subcutaneous injection. Clin Pharm 1992; 11: 347-349.

24. Taddio A, Nulman I, Reid E et al.: Effect of lidocaine-prilocaine cream (EMLA®) on pain of intramuscular Fluzone® injection. Can J Hosp Pharm 1992; 45: 227-230.

25. Taddio A, Nulman I, Goldbach M et al.: Use of lidocaine-prilocaine cream for vaccination pain in infants. J Pediatr 1994; 124: 643-648.

26. Uhari M: A eutectic mixture of lidocaine and prilocaine for alleviating vaccination pain in infants. Pediatrics 1993; 92 (5): 719-721.

9

EMLA Cream for Pain Relief During Arterial Cannulation

Laura A. Magee
The Hospital for Sick Children
Toronto, Ontario, Canada

I. INTRODUCTION

The most common sites for arterial cannulation are the radial and femoral arteries; radial artery cannulation is usually attempted initially. Sites are cannulated percutaneously, usually with a 2-inch, 20-gauge non-tapered Teflon® catheter-over-needle. The indications for arterial line placement can be divided into three broad categories: 1) hemodynamic monitoring (as in a critical care unit or during surgery), 2) serial blood sampling, and 3) intra-arterial administration of drugs.

Arterial cannulation is required in over half of patients admitted to critical care units, many of whom are awake during the insertion process [1]. Other examples of patients requiring arterial line placement include patients with tenuous cardiopulmonary function undergoing major surgery and those undergoing cardiovascular or pulmonary procedures; cannulation usually takes place prior to these procedures. Such surgery is common, and is being done with increasing frequency. For example, in Canada, 10,865 coronary artery bypass operations were performed in 1986–1987, representing a 39% increase over 1981–1982 [2].

EMLA® cream has been shown to produce dermal anesthesia before skin puncture in a variety of circumstances, for example, venipuncture in adults and children [3–5], intravenous catheter insertion in children [6–9], and superficial skin surgery [10]. Percutaneous radial artery cannulation is generally viewed by anesthetists as being more painful than venipuncture; therefore EMLA cream may be useful in this indication. Current practice dictates either premedication of the patient with benzodiazepines or opiates or local infiltration of lidocaine solution (0.5–2%, 0.5 ml); the latter is thought to decrease patient discomfort and decrease the risk of arterial vasospasm. This chapter addresses the potential usefulness of EMLA cream for pain relief prior to arterial cannulation.

II. EFFICACY OF EMLA DURING ARTERIAL CANNULATION

There is every reason to believe that topical application of EMLA cream may be preferable to infiltration with lidocaine. Many believe that local infiltration of anesthetic itself can be quite painful [11], and may increase the perception of pain due to the subsequent procedure [12]. One study found a significant correlation between pain due to needle insertion and that due to intramuscular injection of vaccine, suggesting that the two procedures were not independent [13]. In addition, arterial cannulation may be easier if the vessel is not obscured by infiltrated local anesthetic.

A. Clinical Studies

Three placebo-controlled trials have been published that address the effectiveness of EMLA cream for pain relief during radial arterial cannulation [11,12,14]. EMLA was compared to either placebo cream or infiltration of local anesthetic. In all studies, EMLA cream was administered at a dose of 2.5 g, applied over the radial artery and then covered by an occlusive dressing for a specified period of time (either 60 or 90 minutes). Prior to cannulation, the dressing and emulsion were removed and the skin disinfected. Pain was assessed by the patients and/or a blinded observer using a 10 cm visual analog scale (VAS), ranging from "no pain" to "severe pain." In addition, observer(s) (usually blinded) also rated the patients' pain using a 4-point verbal rating scale (VRS). This ranged from "none" to "severe" pain in two of the studies [12,14], and was scored in the third as: 1 = no response from patient; 2 = mild facial grimace; 3 = verbal response; 4 = withdrawal of hand [11]. There was one observer in two studies [11,12] and two observers in the third study [14]. No study documented intra- or inter-observer variability for these assessments.

Study 1

Smith et al. [11] compared the effectiveness of EMLA to placebo cream and/or lidocaine injection. Forty neurosurgical patients (mean age 48.3; range 22 to 69 years) were enrolled, all of whom had a normal level of consciousness and were without sensory impairment of their upper extremities. Patients were randomly assigned to one of four groups:

1. EMLA cream 60 (i.e., application time at least 60 minutes) alone
2. EMLA cream 60 + saline (0.9%) injection
3. EMLA cream 60 + lidocaine (1%) injection
4. Placebo cream (E35) 60 + lidocaine (1%) injection

The placebo cream appeared similar to EMLA cream when placed under the occlusive dressing. Injections (0.2–0.3 ml solution) were carried out after removal of the occlusive dressing using a 25-gauge needle. The same operator inserted arterial lines in all patients, 2 minutes after infiltration, using a 20-gauge catheter; no information was given on the ease of arterial cannulation.

To assess pain during arterial cannulation, a VAS was completed by all patients (Table 1), and a VRS score noted by one blinded

Table 1 Pain Experience During Arterial Cannulation, Assessed by the Patients Using a Visual Analog Scale

	EMLA applied 60 min	EMLA applied 90 min	EMLA + saline	EMLA + lidocaine	Placebo cream	Lidocaine ± placebo	Statistical difference (p)
Smith et al. [11]						+ Placebo	
No. of patients	10		10	10		10	
Mean scores	25		19.3	27.3		59.1	<0.001[a]
Russell et al. [12]						− Placebo	
No. of patients	20	20				20	
Median scores	30	3.5				22	<0.001[b]
Nilsson et al. [14]							
No. of patients	30				30		
Mean scores	29 ± 26				36 ± 27		NS[c]
No of patients		15			15		
Mean scores		17 ± 28			28 ± 31		NS[c]

[a] All EMLA groups compared to lidocaine infiltration. (Kruskal-Wallis one-way analysis of variance by ranks, and the Mann-Whitney U test.)

[b] EMLA 90 compared to EMLA 60 or lidocaine infiltration. (Mann-Whitney U Test, one-factor analysis of variance for group means.)

[c] NS = not significant. Student's t-test for unpaired data used to compare mean values. This analysis is inappropriate because VAS data are interval; therefore nonparametric tests should be used.

observer (Table 2). The scores were significantly lower on the VAS and VRS for all three EMLA-treated groups compared to the placebo cream-lidocaine infiltration group. There were no significant differences in the VAS or VRS scores between the three EMLA groups.

No serious side effects were noted. Mild blanching was seen in eight of the 30 EMLA patients, versus two of the 10 patients in the placebo cream-lidocaine group; this effect settled within 30 minutes in all patients. Erythema related to the occlusive dressing was observed in three patients (groups not specified).

Study 2

Russell et al. [12] also compared the effectiveness of EMLA cream to lidocaine infiltration. Sixty-four adult patients (mean age 60 ± 9; equal male:female ratio) admitted for elective cardiac surgery were recruited over a 4-month period. Patients were randomly assigned to one of three groups:

1. EMLA cream 60 (application time at least 60 minutes)
2. EMLA cream 90 (application time at least 90 minutes)
3. Lidocaine (2%) injection (2 minutes prior to cannulation, 2 ml solution injected using a 25-gauge needle)

Four EMLA-treated patients were withdrawn because of inadequate placement of the cream; however, the number of patients analyzed in each group was still approximately equal (20, 19, and 20, respectively), which could call into question the randomization process.

Cannulation was accomplished, using a 17.5-gauge catheter, by four different clinicians; however, there was no difference in the mean number of attempts at cannulation. Infiltration with lidocaine did not obscure local anatomy.

Pain was assessed by a VAS completed by the patients (Table 1) and a single, blinded observer; a VRS scale was also completed by the same observer (Table 2). There was no significant difference in VAS or VRS scores between the EMLA 60 group and the lidocaine infiltration group. However, scores were significantly lower on the VAS and the VRS for the EMLA 90 group compared to the other

Table 2 Pain Experience During Arterial Cannulation, Assessed by the Observers Using a 4-Point Verbal Rating Scale

	EMLA applied 60 min	EMLA applied 90 min	EMLA + saline	EMLA + lidocaine	Placebo cream	Lidocaine ± placebo	Statistical difference (p)
Smith et al. [11]						+ placebo	
No. of patients	10		10	10		10	
Mean scores[a]	1.59		11.36	1.59		3.64	<0.001[b]
Russell et al. [12]						− placebo	
No. of patients	20	20				20	
Pain (% per rating)							<0.001[c]
None	15	65				10	
Mild	55	30				40	
Moderate	25	5				45	
Severe	5	0				5	

Nilsson et al. [14]				
No. of patients	30		30	
Pain (% per rating				NS[d]
None	37		26	
Mild	23		20	
Moderate	37		47	
Severe	3		7	
No of patients		15	15	
Pain (% per rating				NS[d]
None		85	62	
Mild		15	8	
Moderate		0	15	
Severe		0	15	

[a] Scores: no response = 0; facial grimace = 2; verbal response = 3; withdrawal from needle = 4.

[b] All EMLA groups compared to lidocaine infiltration. (Kruskal-Wallis one-way analysis of variance by ranks, and the Mann-Whitney U test.)

[c] EMLA 90 compared to EMLA 60 or lidocaine infiltration. (Mann-Whitney U Test, one-factor analysis of variance for group means.)

[d] NS = not significant. Student's t-test for unpaired data used to compare mean values. This analysis is inappropriate because VAS data are interval; therefore nonparametric tests should be used.

two groups. Across all groups, the correlation between observer and patient pain scores was good.

Side effects reported during the study were minimal. Pallor and slight edema at the application site were "common," but "did not persist."

Study 3

Nilsson et al. [14] compared the effectiveness of EMLA to placebo cream in a study involving a total of 90 patients who had been admitted for major surgery for which arterial cannulation was indicated (no demographic data provided). Initially, 60 patients, all of whom had been premedicated with an opiate, were randomly allocated to one of two groups: EMLA cream 60 (application time of 60 minutes) and placebo cream. Cannulation was performed using a Venflon® Arterial Cannula (outer diameter 1 mm); no details are provided on the person(s) responsible for cannulation or on any complications associated with the procedure.

Pain was assessed by completion of a VAS by the patients (Table 1), and a VRS by one of two observing nurses involved in the study (Table 2). (No comment was made on blinding of the observers or inter-observer variability.) There was no significant difference in the VAS or VRS scores when the EMLA 60 group was compared to the placebo cream group. As a result, the investigators decided to study 30 additional patients, following the same protocol, with random allocation to the following groups: 1) EMLA cream 90 (application time of 90 minutes) and 2) placebo cream.

Results were reported for 13 patients in each of the two groups; there were four drop-outs, due to either failure to perform arterial cannulation or cancellation of surgery. With this extended application time of 90 minutes, there was no statistically significant difference in the VAS scores for pain (Table 1); however, the VRS scores were significantly lower in the EMLA 90 group (Table 2).

No side effects of clinical importance were observed, although pallor or erythema at the site of application was noted (frequency not given).

III. DISCUSSION

The three randomized, placebo-controlled trials of EMLA cream, done in diverse groups of adult patients, arrived at a similar conclusion: EMLA cream is effective in decreasing pain associated with arterial cannulation. Two studies reported EMLA to be superior to placebo cream and/or local anesthesia, based on VAS and VRS scores, when EMLA cream was applied for "at least" 60 to 90 minutes before cannulation [11,12]. The third study reported EMLA superiority only after an application time of 90 minutes, based only on VRS scores [14]; however, this study was methodologically the weakest, and the statistical analyses of the data were not appropriate.

It is not surprising that EMLA cream may need to be applied for a more prolonged period of time prior to arterial, as opposed to venous, cannulation. Although EMLA cream has been shown to penetrate intact skin and produce reliable cutaneous anesthesia after 45 to 60 minutes of application [5], it should be noted that cutaneous pain sensation is conducted not only by superficial fast myelinated A fibers, but also by deeper slow unmyelinated C fibers; the latter are the predominant innervation of the subcutaneous tissue and vessel wall. Ray and Wolff [15], in observing neurosurgical patients, noted that extracranial arteries were more sensitive to pain than veins, and anesthesia was obtained by introduction of procaine hydrochloride into the adventitia of the artery; the implication was that sensory nerves travel along with the arteries. Consistent with this is the observation that, for the purposes of pain relief for superficial skin surgery, EMLA cream must be applied for 120 minutes [10]. Therefore, before arterial puncture, it would seem that one needs to allow at least 60 to 90 minutes for EMLA cream to penetrate the deeper tissues.

It is interesting to note that the VAS scores reported for the three studies were quite different. Some of the discrepancy may be accounted for by reporting of median versus mean scores, although only if the data were skewed. EMLA 60 produced fairly similar average VAS scores of 30 [12], 29 ± 26 [14] and 25 [11]. However, despite the fact all patients had been admitted for elective surgery, EMLA 90 scores in the two studies using this application time were quite different: 3.5 [12] and 17 ± 28 [14]. This occurred despite the fact that the patients in the latter study received premedication with opiate. Insufficient information was presented regarding the details of the cannulation procedure [11,14] to comment on differences. In addition, there are many other variables that affect the amount of pain perceived by patients, so the comparability of the raw scores is in question.

It should be noted, however, that such discrepancies in VAS scores may relate to differences in cannulation technique or the unreliability of the assessment (VAS and VRS) used to measure pain. The methodology used for future studies should address these possibilities, and include pre-testing of the VAS to ensure understanding.

It is not surprising that side effects occurring with EMLA cream consisted of mild, temporary blanching or erythema of the skin. None was considered serious.

IV. CONCLUSION

The evidence to date supports the efficacy of EMLA cream in decreasing pain in the patient who has not been premedicated prior to arterial cannulation. However, the required application time would seem to be 60 to 90 minutes, i.e. longer than that needed for venipuncture. It should be noted that only small numbers of patients have been assessed to date. Future research should ensure use of a reliable method for the measurement of pain, compare the effectiveness of EMLA cream to premedication prior to arterial cannulation, and address the issues of patient preference and cost.

REFERENCES

1. Seneff M: Arterial line placement and care. In: Atlas of Procedures in the Intensive Care Unit. pp 37-47.
2. Peters S et al.: Coronary artery bypass surgery in Canada. Health Reports 1990; 2(1): 9-26.
3. Wahlstedt C, Kollberg H, Moller C: Lignocaine-prilocaine cream reduces venipuncture pain. Lancet 1984; 14: 106.

4. Hallen B, Carlsson P, Uppfeldt A: Clinical study of a lignocaine-prilocaine cream to relieve the pain of venipuncture. Br J Anaesth 1985; 57: 326-328.

5. Ehrenstrom-Reiz G, Reiz S, Stockman O: Topical anaesthesia with EMLA, a new lidocaine-prilocaine cream and the cusum technique for detection of minimal application time. Acta Anaesthesiol Scand 1983; 27: 510-512.

6. Hopkins CS, Buckley CJ, Bush GH: Pain-free injection in infants; use of a lignocaine-prilocaine cream to prevent pain at intravenous induction of general anaesthesia in 1–5 year old children. Anaesthesia 1988; 43: 198-201.

7. Soliman IE, Broadman LM, Hannallah RS, McGill WA: Comparison of the analgesic effects of EMLA (eutectic mixture of local anaesthetics) to intradermal lidocaine infiltration prior to venous cannulation in unpremedicated children. Anesthesiology 1988; 68: 804-806.

8. Hallen B, Olsson GL, Uppfeldt A: Pain-free venepuncture; effect of timing of application of local anaesthetic cream. Anaesthesia 1984; 39: 969-972.

9. Hallen B, Uppfeldt A: Does lidocaine-prilocaine cream permit pain-free insertion of IV catheters in children? Anesthesiology 1982; 57: 340-342.

10. Juhlin L, Broberg F: A lidocaine-prilocaine cream for superficial skin surgery and painful lesions. Acta Derm Venereol 1980; 60: 544-546.

11. Smith M, Gray BM, Ingram S, Jewkes DA: Double-blind comparison to topical lignocaine-prilocaine cream (EMLA) and lignocaine infiltration for arterial cannulation in adults. Br J of Anaesthesiol 1990; 65: 240-242.

12. Russell GN, Desmond MJ, Fox MA: Local anesthesia for radial artery cannulation: A comparison of a lidocaine-prilocaine emulsion and lidocaine infiltration. J Cardiothor Anesth 1988; 2(3): 309-312.

13. Taddio A et al.: Effect of lidocaine-prilocaine cream (EMLA) on pain of intramuscular fluzone injection. Can J Hosp Pharm 1992; 45: 227-30.

14. Nilsson A et al.: EMLA for pain relief during arterial cannulation. Upsala J Med 1990; 95: 87-94.

15. Ray BS, Wolff HG: Experimental studies on headache. Arch Surg 1940; 41: 813-856.

10

Use of EMLA Cream in Dermatosurgical Interventions of Skin and Genital Mucosa

Arnold P. Oranje and Flora B. de Waard-van der Spek

University Hospital Rotterdam—Sophia
Rotterdam, The Netherlands

I. INTRODUCTION

EMLA® cream has been shown to induce topical analgesia for a number of superficial skin interventions [1,2]. For example, EMLA analgesia has been successfully used in curettage of molluscum contagiosum, in cauterization of condylomata acuminata and in laser therapy of port-wine stains. This chapter reviews studies on the use of EMLA cream for these dermatosurgical interventions of skin and genital mucosa.

II. MOLLUSCUM CONTAGIOSUM

Molluscum contagiosum is a benign skin tumor caused by a large poxvirus. The disease is self-limiting, but intercurrent infection and its cosmetic unacceptability make treatment desirable. Treatment consists of curettage or brief application of liquid nitrogen; application of etching creams or lotions is less effective. Curettage of molluscum contagiosum is painful and distressing, especially when multiple lesions (more than five) are present, and it is very common to find 10 to 20 mollusca per individual. In the past, curettage of more than 30 mollusca was often performed under general anesthesia. However, it is now considered desirable to avoid general anesthesia whenever possible, especially because more than one treatment is often necessary.

A. Clinical Studies

A preliminary study by Juhlin [3] reported results in eight children, in whom sufficient analgesia was observed using EMLA cream with an application time of 30 to 45 minutes.

de Waard-van der Spek et al. [4] carried out a double-blind, placebo-controlled, study in 83 children, aged 4 to 12 years, each with at least five mollusca. The main aim of the study was to assess the efficacy and minimal effective application time of EMLA cream for the curettage of molluscum contagiosum. Patients were randomly assigned to receive either EMLA ($n = 58$) or placebo ($n = 25$) cream, applied for 15, 30 or 60 minutes before curettage. Pain was assessed by the patients using both a 4-point verbal rating scale (VRS) and a visual analog scale (VAS), and by the physicians using the verbal scale. The patients' and physicians' assessments were in agreement and showed that application of EMLA cream for all three periods significantly reduced the pain ($p < 0.01$). Although there was no significant difference observed between the 15-, 30- and 60-minute groups, the frequency of "no pain" increased from 36% in the 15-minute group to 61% in the 60-minute group. Overall, 87% of the children treated with EMLA cream compared to 52% of the children in the placebo group felt either no pain or only slight pain. This difference was statistically significant.

Wagner and Mensing [5] studied the use of EMLA cream in an open study involving 40 children, aged 2 to 11 years, with multiple mollusca contagiosa (5 to 42 per child). EMLA cream was applied for 30 minutes before curettage. None of the children complained of pain during curettage.

Rosdahl et al. [6] reported an open study involving 55 children, aged 3 to 14 years. Five to 25 mollusca per child were covered with a maximum of 10 g EMLA cream, 1 hour before curettage. Pain was rated on a VAS, in which 0 mm denoted "no pain" and 100 mm denoted "maximal pain," by both the patient and the investigator. No pain or only slight pain was felt by 93% (children's assessment) or 96% (physician's assessment) of the patients treated with EMLA cream. The median rating on the VAS was 3 mm.

EMLA cream (30-minute application time) has also been show to be effective in providing analgesia for the removal of molluscum by brief application of liquid nitrogen. However, this method of removal is not applicable to dark-skinned subjects, and is less controlled than curettage.

III. CONDYLOMATA ACUMINATA

Condylomata acuminata (CA) are anogenital warts that are widespread in adolescents and adults. The infection, which is caused by human papillomaviruses (HPV), is usually sexually transmitted. To date, about 60 HPV types have been identified, but only some of these are responsible for CA infections [7]. Condylomata acuminata have also been reported in children [8,9]. CA are removed by cauterization or laser treatment, and the efficacy of EMLA analgesia during this treatment has been investigated in a number of clinical studies.

A. Clinical Studies

A preliminary study by Hallen et al. [10], suggested that EMLA cream provided effective analgesia for the cautery of genital warts in 96% ($n = 57$) of men but only 40 % of the 51 women in the study. However, a later study by Ljunghall and Lillieborg [11] found that EMLA cream was effective on vulval mucosa provided that the application time was optimized. Ten women were enrolled in a pilot study for establishing the time of onset of analgesia, as determined by a pinch test. Anesthesia was found to occur after application times of only 5 to 7 minutes. A further 42 women underwent cautery of genital warts following application of EMLA cream for 10, 15 or 20 minutes. A 10-minute application provided sufficient anesthesia for the cautery of genital warts in 92% of the women. However, longer application times resulted in less effective analgesia [11], which may explain the apparent failure of EMLA cream to provide adequate analgesia in studies where EMLA was applied to female genital mucosa for longer periods.

Rylander et al. [12] assessed the time of onset and application time required for EMLA-induced local anesthesia, in a double-blind trial involving 80 women with CA on the genital mucosa. EMLA ($n = 60$) or placebo ($n = 20$) cream was applied 1 to 75 minutes prior to carbon dioxide laser treatment of a test site containing a CA lesion. The degree of pain experienced was assessed by the patient using a VAS. Analgesia was discernible after only 4 to 5 minutes, although the most effective analgesia was achieved after applying EMLA cream for 5 to 15 minutes. Patients given EMLA cream, regardless of application time, recorded significantly lower pain scores than the placebo group. Additional analgesia was required for seven patients (12%) in the EMLA-treated group and for all 20 patients in the placebo-treated group.

Van den Berg et al. [13], in an open study of 60 men, compared the analgesic efficacy achieved by EMLA cream and by lidocaine injection for punch biopsy and electrocoagulation of CA on the genital area and/or perianal area. EMLA cream ($n = 31$) was applied for 13 to 45 minutes, or lidocaine infiltration ($n = 29$) carried out 0.5 to 4 minutes prior to removal of the warts by electrocoagulation. Pain was assessed by the patient using a 4-point VRS and a VAS. Lidocaine injection itself was reported to be slightly (59% of patients) or moderately (34%) painful, whereas application of EMLA cream was painless. EMLA cream had a lower analgesic efficacy than lidocaine infiltration for electrocoagulation (satisfactory analgesia achieved in 62% vs. 100% of patients, respectively), but EMLA cream proved very useful for taking punch biopsies (effective analgesia achieved in 94% of patients) or as premedication to alleviate the pain of infiltration.

A similar study, comparing EMLA cream (application time 10 minutes) with lidocaine infiltration, was carried out by Lassus et al. [14]. This study assessed the pain experienced during administration of anesthesia and during laser surgery of genital warts in 100 male patients. Although the efficacy of infiltrated anesthetic was slightly better than EMLA cream in alleviating pain during surgery, the overall treatment (administration and surgery) pain score was significantly lower in the EMLA group, as a result of the higher pain scores for the infiltration process. The authors therefore suggested that EMLA cream should be the treatment of choice in laser surgery of genital warts.

A more recent study by Frega et al. [15] also recommended EMLA cream as the anesthetic of choice for laser surgery of genital warts. Pain during administration of anesthesia and during surgery was assessed in 180 patients (90 males and 90 females) receiving EMLA cream and 90 patients (45 males and 45 females) receiving 2% Carbocaine® infiltration. The application time for EMLA cream was 5 to 18 minutes (median 7 minutes). Unlike the study of Lassus et al. [14], results from this study indicated that pain was significantly less in the EMLA group than in the infiltration group both during administration of anesthesia and during laser surgery. Side effects of pallor and/or edema occurred more often in the infiltration group; this together with occasional bleeding could affect the efficacy of laser treatment.

IV. BIOPSIES

For skin biopsies, it is important to provide analgesia to a sufficient skin depth (i.e., optimize application time), as pain may be felt in the dermis if deep biopsies are taken [2]. The maximum depth of analgesia provided by EMLA cream is reported to be about 5 mm [16], which should be sufficient for taking skin biopsies. Thune et al. [17] reported an open study comparing the efficacy of EMLA cream or prilocaine infiltration anesthesia in 51 patients requiring punch or excision skin biopsy. The duration of EMLA cream application ranged from 60 to 195 minutes (mean 121 minutes). There were no significant differences between the VAS pain scores of the patients who received EMLA cream ($n = 34$) and those who received injection ($n = 17$), and the authors concluded that, used appropriately, EMLA cream provides effective local anesthesia for taking skin biopsies.

Byrne et al. [18] obtained vulval biopsies from 10 female patients after applying EMLA cream for 15 to 20 minutes (somewhat longer than the optimal application time for vulval mucosa). The results showed that 88% of the biopsies were successfully anesthetized; two patients required additional analgesia. A similar success rate was observed in male patients by Van den Berg et al. [13], who found that EMLA cream provided effective analgesia for punch biopsy on the genital/perianal area of 95% of male patients ($n = 31$) when applied for 13 to 45 minutes.

Ogborn [19] reported an open study of eight non-sedated children undergoing renal biopsy. EMLA cream was used to anesthetize the area through which incision, deep infiltration of 2% lidocaine and biopsy with 18- or 14-gauge needles was carried out. All patients cooperated well with the procedure; only three reported mild discomfort during the initial puncture. The author concluded that EMLA cream was useful in improving the speed and comfort of renal biopsies.

V. INFILTRATION PAIN

Virtually all clinical trials that have compared the pain associated with administration of EMLA cream with that experienced on infiltration of local anesthetics report a relatively high level of pain during the infiltration procedure. Some of these trials have involved supplementation of EMLA analgesia with infiltration anesthesia. In most cases, the pain experienced during infiltration into EMLA-treated skin was said to be less than that normally experienced in unanesthetized skin. However, clinical studies specifically designed to investigate the use of EMLA cream as a premedication to alleviate pain during infiltration have produced conflicting results.

A study by Zilbert and Lewandowski [20] investigated the analgesic efficacy of EMLA cream prior to infiltration of a lidocaine 1% solution in the vulval mucosa. EMLA ($n = 21$) or placebo ($n = 23$)

cream was applied over the vulva 6 to 10 minutes before infiltration of lidocaine, then the degree of pain experienced during infiltration was noted by the patients on a 100 mm VAS and 4-point VRS. The mean VAS score for EMLA cream was 23.4 mm, compared to 43.0 mm for the placebo ($p < 0.005$). Verbal ratings of moderate or severe pain were given by 23.8% of EMLA-treated patients, compared to 52.2% of those given placebo. The authors concluded that EMLA provided effective analgesia for local anesthetic infiltration of the vulva, a procedure that can be particularly painful in this sensitive area of the body.

Jones et al. [21] reported a double-blind, placebo-controlled study in which EMLA or placebo cream was used as premedication for percutaneous lidocaine infiltration. A total of 65 patients undergoing minor skin surgery were divided into two groups, the first group having one lesion and the second group having two lesions. The first group was randomized to receive either EMLA or placebo cream as premedication, the second group received EMLA on one lesion and placebo on the other. In contrast to the results of Zilbert and Lewand-owski [20] in vulval mucosa, Jones et al. found that EMLA cream applied for 1 hour was not particularly effective in eliminating pain caused by local-anesthetic injection in normal skin.

VI. PORT-WINE STAINS

In the past, the use of argon and carbon dioxide lasers for removal of port-wine stains resulted in very painful operations, and infiltration of lidocaine to alleviate the laser pain was in itself painful. In addition, argon lasers could cause scarring and were not very effective in pale port-wine stains. The more recently available pulsed-dye laser can be used for pale port-wine stains and is less painful than treatment with other types of lasers. Thus, this type of laser therapy is now available for young children.

Lasers have been used in models to compare the efficacy of different anesthetics. For example, Arendt-Nielsen and Bjerring [22] reported a study in which the efficacy of EMLA cream was compared with that of lidocaine infiltration, using an argon laser for experimental pain stimulation. Three parameters were measured: pain threshold (i.e., when no pain was felt but other sensations could be detected), sensory threshold (no sensations felt) and pain-related cortical responses. The effect of EMLA cream application time on the efficacy and duration of analgesia was determined. With application times of less than 2 hours, the analgesic effect of EMLA increased after removal of the cream. Lidocaine infiltration provided total sensory block almost immediately after injection. A similar degree of efficacy was given by EMLA cream, either immediately after an application time of 100 or 120 minutes or 20 minutes after removal of the cream following an application time of 80 minutes.

A. Clinical Studies

Several studies on the clinical use of EMLA cream for the treatment of port-wine stains with pulsed-dye lasers have been reported (see below). These have shown that EMLA provides pain-free administration of effective analgesia without affecting the degree of lightening of the port-wine stain achieved during treatment.

Lanigan and Cotterill [23] reported the effect of EMLA cream in the treatment of facial port-wine stains with a tunable dye laser. The cream provided adequate analgesia in eight of the 10 patients treated, and was well tolerated. The results of the laser treatment were no different in the EMLA group compared to those given conventional infiltration analgesia, and the authors concluded that EMLA cream could be recommended for use during port-wine stain removal.

Ashihnoff and Geronemus [24] investigated whether pretreatment with EMLA cream, which is thought to cause vasoconstriction of cutaneous blood vessels, affects the efficacy of subsequent pulsed-dye laser treatment of port-wine stains. Eight patients, aged 4 to 32 years, received test treatments on two sites in the same area of port-wine stain. One of the sites was pretreated with EMLA cream (60 minutes application under occlusion followed by 15 minutes unoccluded); the other site was not pretreated. EMLA cream was found to provide effective topical analgesia during treatment. Examination of the test sites 6 to 8 weeks after laser treatment showed that EMLA pretreatment did not affect the degree of lightening of the port-wine stain. Thus

EMLA cream can be used to alleviate the pain of laser dye treatment without affecting the efficacy of removal of the port-wine stain.

Tan and Stafford [25] assessed the efficacy of EMLA cream vs. placebo or no treatment in a study involving 73 children (aged 5 to 16 years) treated with pulsed-dye laser for port-wine stain. Three test sites within one area of port-wine stain were pretreated with EMLA cream, placebo cream or no cream, and covered with an occlusive dressing for 60 minutes. Laser treatment was then carried out on each area and the degree of pain experienced assessed by the patient, physician and an independent observer, using a modified VAS that included diagrams ranging from happy to crying faces. The pain scores for the three individuals carrying out the assessments were in good agreement. The mean pain scores for no treatment, placebo and EMLA were 38.6, 32.1 and 10.9, respectively. These values were significantly different from one another ($p < 0.0001$). The investigators also reported that 52% of the EMLA-treated sites were pain-free during laser therapy, compared with only 11% of placebo-treated sites ($p < 0.001$).

VII. OTHER INDICATIONS

A. Acne

Whiteheads, a common symptom in acne, not only are disfiguring but may also develop into painful inflamed lesions. Application of EMLA cream for 60 to 180 minutes has been shown to provide adequate pain relief for such inflamed lesions [26].

A study reported by Bottomley et al. [27] used EMLA cream during light electrocautery and fulguration of whiteheads in 12 patients. The pain scores (VAS) varied considerably between individuals in the study. One patient who was unable to tolerate either electrocautery or fulguration without analgesia was found to tolerate fulguration when EMLA was provided.

B. Hirsutism

All the currently available methods for hair removal, such as electrolysis, thermolysis and temporary methods (e.g., wax) cause pain or discomfort during the procedure. Induction of analgesia by infiltration can be very painful in some areas of the face, such as the upper lip, where excess hair is commonly located. The use of EMLA cream in epilation therefore has great potential. Only one clinical trial has been reported to date. Hjorth et al. [28] investigated 21 patients in a double-blind, placebo-controlled cross-over study. EMLA or placebo cream (5 g) was applied to the upper lip for 1 hour, then hair was removed by thermolysis over a period of 10 minutes. Pain was assessed by the subject and the cosmetologist on a 4-point scale. Significantly less pain was experienced with EMLA compared to placebo, and 90% of the patients expressed a preference for EMLA cream.

C. Common Warts

A study reported by Vesterager et al. [29] showed that EMLA cream does not provide effective analgesia for the removal of common warts by curettage. A total of 89 patients were evaluated; 47 received lidocaine infiltration and 42 received EMLA cream (2.5 g, 120 minutes application time). Although the pain rating for administration of anesthetic was significantly lower for the EMLA group (100% reported "no pain," compared to 25% in the lidocaine group), the overall rating for EMLA was significantly less than that for lidocaine ("very good" overall impression reported by 33% and 62% of patients, respectively; $p < 0.001$) owing to the less effective analgesia provided during curettage. The efficacy of EMLA did not depend on the size of the wart. The results suggest that EMLA does not penetrate the highly hyperkeratotic wart area at a rate sufficient to allow accumulation of EMLA in the skin, and the authors concluded that EMLA could not be recommended for curettage of warts.

Oranje and de Waard-van der Spek (unpublished observation) have also noted that EMLA analgesia is not sufficient for the removal of common warts by the process of cryotreatment.

D. Adenoma Sebaceum

Satisfactory results were obtained with EMLA cream (application time 60 minutes) by Oranje and de Waard-van der Spek (unpublished data) in studies in which a carbon dioxide laser was used to treat adults with adenoma sebaceum.

VIII. SIDE EFFECTS

Many patients develop local redness or pallor of the skin of brief duration, but no major side effects have been reported with the correct use of EMLA cream. One case of vesicles at the site of an EMLA dressing and three occurrences of purpura at the EMLA cream application site have been recorded by Oranje and de Waard-van der Spek (unpublished observation). Purpura was noted in patients with atopic dermatitis in the groin or axilla.

IX. CONCLUSION

Used correctly, EMLA cream is a safe and effective topical anesthetic. Application times required for the cream range from about 10 minutes for mucous membranes to 2 hours for the skin. The main indications are curettage of molluscum contagiosum, cauterization of condylomata acuminata, laser therapy of port-wine stains and superficial surgical procedures at the mucous membranes (see Table 1). EMLA cream can also be used as premedication for lidocaine infiltration, although successful analgesia has not always been achieved in this indication.

It is justified to conclude that this analgesic cream is a very welcome addition for use in different superficial surgical interventions.

Table 1 Applications of EMLA Cream in Superficial Skin Conditions

Indication	Application time (min)	Most relevant ref.
Molluscum contagiosum	15–30	de Waard-van der Spek et al. [4]
Condylomata acuminata	5–20	Rylander et al. [11]
Port-wine stains	60	Arendt-Nielsen and Bjerring [17]

REFERENCES

1. de Waard-van der Spek FB, Berg van den GM, Oranje AP: EMLA Cream: an improved local anesthetic. Review of current literature. Pediatr Dermatol 1992; 9: 126-131.

2. Juhlin L, Evers H: EMLA: a new topical anesthetic. Adv Dermatol 1990; 5: 75-92.

3. Juhlin L, Evers H, Broberg F: A lidocaine-prilocaine cream for superficial skin surgery and painful lesions. Acta Dermatovener 1980; 60: 544-546.

4. de Waard-van der Spek FB, Oranje AP, Lillieborg S, et al.: Treatment of molluscum contagiosum under analgesia with a lidocaine/prilocaine cream (EMLA). J Am Acad Dermatol 1990; 23: 685-688.

5. Wagner G, Mensing H: Erfahrungen mit der perkutanen Anasthesie bei Verwendung einer Lidocain-Prilocain-Creme (EMLA Cream® 5%). Zeitschrift Hautkrankh 1989; 64: 688-693.

6. Rosdahl I, Edmar B, Gisslen H, et al.: Curettage of molluscum contagiosum in children: Analgesia by topical application of a lidocaine/prilocaine cream (EMLA). Acta Derm Venereol (Stockh) 1988; 68: 149-153.

7. Chuang TY: Condylomata acuminata (genital warts): epidemiologic view. J Am Acad Dermatol 1987; 16: 376-384.

8. Oranje AP, de Waard-van der Spek FB, Vuzevski VD, et al.: Condylomata acuminata in children. Int J STD AIDS 1990; 1: 250-255.

9. Davis AD, Emans J: Human papilloma virus infection in the pediatric and adolescent patient. J Pediatr 1989; 115: 1-9.

10. Hallen A, Ljunghall K, Wallin J: Topical anaesthesia with local anaesthetic (lidocaine and prilocaine, EMLA) cream for cautery of genital warts. Genitourin Med 1987; 63: 316-319.

11. Ljunghall K, Lillieborg S: Local anaesthesia with a lidocaine/prilocaine cream (EMLA) for cautery of condylomata acuminata on the vulvar mucosa. The effect of timing of application of the cream. Acta Derm Venereol (Stockh) 1989; 69: 362-365.

12. Rylander E, Sjoberg I, Lillieborg S, Stockman O: Local anaesthesia of the genital mucosa with a lidocaine/prilocaine cream (EMLA) for laser treatment of condylomata acuminata: a placebo-controlled study. Obstet Gynecol 1990; 75: 302-306.

13. van den Berg GM, Lillieborg S, Stolz E: Lidocaine/prilocaine cream (EMLA®) versus infiltration anaesthesia: a comparison of the analgesic efficacy for punch biopsy and electrocoagulation of genital warts in men. Genitourin Med 1992; 68: 162-165.

14. Lassus A, Kartamaa M, Happonen H-P: A comparative study of topical analgesia with a lidocaine/prilocaine cream (EMLA) and infiltration anaesthesia for laser surgery of genital warts in men. Sex Trasmit Dis 1990; 17: 130-132.

15. Frega A, Di Renzi F, Palazzetti PL, Pace S, Figliolini M, Stentella P: Vulvar and penile HPV lesions: laser surgery and topical anaesthesia. Clin Exp Obstet Gynecol 1993; 20(2): 76-81.

16. Bjerring P, Arendt-Nielsen L: Depth and duration of skin analgesia to needle insertion after topical application of EMLA cream. Br J Anaesth 1990; 64: 173-177.

17. Thune P, Faerden F, Minor BG: The analgesic effect of EMLA® cream for skin biopsies. J Dermatol Treat 1990; 1: 239-241.

18. Byrne MA, Taylor-Robinson D, Harris JRW: Topical anaesthesia with lidocaine/prilocaine cream for vulval biopsy. Br J Obstet Gynaecol 1989; 96: 497-500.

19. Ogborn MR: The use of a eutectic mixture of local anesthetic in pediatric renal biopsy. Pediatr Nephrol 1992; 6: 276-277.

20. Zilbert AW, Lewandowski K: The analgesic effect of lidocaine-prilocaine cream proir to infiltration anaesthesia of the vulva. Nova Scotia Med J December 1993; 210-211.

21. Jones SK, Handfield-Jones S, Kennedy CTC: Does EMLA reduce the discomfort associated with local-anaesthetic infiltration? Clin Exp Dermatol 1990; 15: 177-179.

22. Arendt-Nielsen L, Bjerring P: Laser-induced pain for evaluation of local analgesia: a comparison of topical application (EMLA) and local injections (lidocaine). Anesth Analg 1988; 67: 115-123.

23. Lanigan SW, Cotterill JA: Use of a lignocaine/prilocaine cream as an analgesic in dye laser treatment of port-wine stains. Lasers Med Sci 1987; 2: 87-89.

24. Ashinhoff R, Geronemus RG: Effect of the topical anesthetic EMLA on the efficacy of pulsed dye laser treatment of port-wine stains. J Dermatol Surg Oncol 1990; 16: 1008-1011.

25. Tan OT, Stafford TJ: EMLA for laser treatment of port-wine stains in children. Lasers Surg Med 1992; 12: 543-548.

26. Pepall LM, Cosgrove MP, Cunliffe WJ: Ablation of whiteheads by cautery under topical anaesthesia. Br J Dermatol 1991; 125: 256-259.
27. Bottomley WW, Yip J, Knaggs H, Cunliffe WJ: Treatment of closed comedones: comparisons of fulguration with topical tretinoin and electrocautery with fulguration. Dermatology 1993; 186: 253-257.
28. Hjorth N, Harring M, Hahn A: Epilation of upper lip hirsutism with a eutectic mixture of lidocaine and prilocaine used as a topical local anesthetic. J Am Acad Dermatol 1991; 25: 809-811.
29. Vesterager L, Pfeiffer Petersen K, Nielsen R, Niordson AM, Gammeltoft M, Graudal C, Stahl D: EMLA-induced analgesia inferior to lidocaine infiltration in curettage of common warts: a randomised study. Dermatology 1994; 188: 32-35.

11

Use of EMLA Sterile Cream in the Management of Leg Ulcers

Donald Rosenthal

McMaster University
Hamilton, Ontario, Canada

I. INTRODUCTION

It is well recognized that the number of older people is increasing in the general population, and it is members of this age group who are most prone to the development of leg ulcers. While the etiology of leg ulcers is often multifactorial, vascular insufficiency is the most common underlying factor. Thus, as the population ages, the prevalence of chronic leg ulcers of vascular origin will increase. Callam [1] has estimated that 17% of the population of the United Kingdom will eventually develop a chronic leg ulcer. Anderson et al. [2] concluded that the prevalence of leg and feet ulcers in Sweden is 0.2 to 0.4% of all adults and up to 2% in the older age group, with equal distribution between men and women.

Despite the availability of physical and surgical interventions, multiple dressings and oral medications, the management of patients with chronic vascular induced leg ulcers is often frustrating, time-consuming, costly and unrewarding. Surgical debridement is often used in the treatment of chronic leg ulcers, in an attempt to define the ulcer depth and to achieve "cleaner areas" that will granulate and heal more effectively. However, the process is frequently painful and the availability of topical anesthesia should greatly benefit patients receiving such treatment.

This chapter reviews the use of EMLA® sterile cream for the analgesia and management of leg ulcers as reported in recent literature.

II. CLINICAL STUDIES

While all studies involving the use of EMLA sterile cream in leg ulcers have covered both safety and efficacy aspects, they have been categorized here into those that report mainly on plasma levels, those that assess efficacy, and trials involving repeated use.

A. Plasma Levels of Lidocaine and Prilocaine

Study 1

Larsson-Stymne et al. [3] performed an open clinical study of plasma concentrations of lidocaine and prilocaine after prolonged application of EMLA sterile cream to leg ulcers. Ten patients (median age 79 years, range 71 to 86) with venous, arteriovenous or arterial ulcers took part in this study. A layer of EMLA sterile cream (1 g/10 cm^2) was applied to ulcers with areas of between 50 and 100 cm^2, for 24 hours. Venous blood samples were obtained prior to and up to 24 or 27 hours after application.

Maximum plasma concentrations were observed at 2 to 4 hours and ranged between 185 and 705 ng/ml for lidocaine and 62 and 277 ng/ml for prilocaine. Three patients reported slight or moderate burning sensation, two patients exhibited erythema and one patient had edema, pallor and erythema. The authors concluded that prolonged application of EMLA sterile cream at a dose of 5 to 10 g to leg ulcers resulted in plasma concentrations far below toxic levels (which are 5000 to 6000 ng/ml), and side effects were minimal.

Study 2

Enander-Malmros et al. [4] conducted a two-part study, the first part of which assessed plasma concentrations of lidocaine and prilocaine in eight patients with ulcers of venous, arterial, arteriovenous or immunological origin. Patients were aged 60 to 83 years (median 74 years), with leg ulcers of area 31 to 80 cm^3 and duration 1 to 10 years. A non-standard preparation of sterile EMLA cream containing 2% anesthetic, rather than the standard 5%, was applied for 60 minutes at a dose of 1.2 to 2.8 g cream per 10 cm^2 ulcer. Blood samples were obtained for analysis before application of the cream and at 30-minute intervals between 1 and 4 hours afterward. The lowest sensitivity of the assay was 10 ng/ml for both lidocaine and prilocaine.

The highest individual plasma concentrations of the anesthetic agents detected were 205 ng/ml lidocaine in a patient with an arterial ulcer measuring 56 cm^2 and 79 ng/ml prilocaine in a patient with an arteriovenous ulcer measuring 37 cm^2. No systemic adverse reactions were observed, and, as in other studies, plasma concentrations of lidocaine and prilocaine were 20 to 35 times lower than those associated with toxicity (5000 to 6000 ng/ml). Adverse effects reported were a slight (one patient) or severe (one patient) burning sensation and slight local pallor (one patient).

In two patients with arterial or arteriovenous ulcers, the maximal concentrations (C_{max}) were observed after 60 minutes. However, in patients with venous disease or rheumatoid arthritis, maximal concentrations were reached at 120 and 90 minutes, respectively. In patients with ulcers of arterial origin, the peak concentration of lidocaine/prilocaine may be reached earlier due to a decreased absorption rate secondary to impaired venous return. The C_{max} of lidocaine tended to increase with increasing ulcer area, but this was not the case with prilocaine.

B.   Efficacy During Debridement

Study 1

Holm and co-workers [5] investigated the analgesic effect of EMLA sterile cream on the debridement of leg ulcers. This was done in both an open study and a double-blind placebo-controlled comparison involving 80 patients with ulcers of arterial or venous origin. The size of the ulcers varied between 24 and 64 cm^2, and their duration varied from 1 month to 38 years. EMLA sterile cream or placebo (5 or 10 g) was applied 10 to 30 minutes prior to debridement. Blood samples were collected before and up to 3 hours after (at 30-minute intervals) application of the cream, for analysis of plasma concentrations of lidocaine and prilocaine. The analgesic effect was assessed on a 4-point verbal scale ranging from none to severe and a 100 mm visual analog scale (VAS). For each patient, the investigator assessed whether the debridement was satisfactory.

The plasma concentrations of the anesthetic agents were reported to be much lower than those classically associated with toxicity. The median VAS pain score for the EMLA treated group was statistically lower than that for the placebo group. The debridement was judged satisfactory in the majority of patients in the EMLA group and in a reduced number in the placebo group. A transient burning sensation was noted by 15% of EMLA patients while a very small number of the placebo patients reported a similar sensation. The authors stated that they could detect no untoward effects on ulcer healing due to application of EMLA sterile cream and concluded that local anesthesia with topical EMLA offered the majority of patients statistically and clinically good pain relief compared to placebo.

Study 2

In a recently completed double-blind, placebo-controlled trial [6], 101 patients aged between 29 and 99 years (median 72), all of whom were scheduled for mechanical debridement of a chronic leg ulcer, were enrolled at four Canadian dermatology centers. All patients enrolled into this study had experienced pain associated with a previous debridement. Sixty-one patients were assessed as having leg ulcers primarily of venous origin, 12 patients had ulcers of arterial origin and 26 were of mixed arterial venous origin. A thick layer of EMLA or placebo was applied to the ulcer under occlusion for 30 minutes. The pain experienced during subsequent debridement was rated by both the patient and the investigator on a 100 mm VAS.

Statistically less pain was experienced by the EMLA group than by the placebo group. No systemic adverse reactions were noted in any of the patients. Mild, transient redness, pallor or edema was noted by 16% of the patients in the EMLA group and 20% of the patients in the placebo group. The authors concluded that, if applied appropriately, EMLA sterile cream can significantly reduce the pain associated with debridement of chronic, vascular-induced leg ulcers.

C. Repeated Use of EMLA

Study 1

In the second part of the investigation by Enander-Malmros et al. [4], the efficacy of repeat applications of two concentrations of EMLA (2% or 5%) was assessed in a double-blind, four-period, cross-over study. 2% or 5% EMLA cream was randomly applied to 10 patients for 30 minutes before four consecutive cleansings, 1 to 4 days apart (each patient received both concentrations twice during the four treatments). The dose of cream was 0.75 to 9.0 g (median 2.9 g) per 10 cm^2 of ulcer. A 100 mm VAS and a 4-point verbal scale were used for pain evaluation.

The analgesic effect was similar for the 2% and 5% EMLA cream; in 80 to 90% of treatments the patient felt no or slight pain during cleansing. However, the post-cleansing pain tended to be higher with 2% than with 5% EMLA cream, indicating a possible difference in duration of anesthesia. The pain experienced during the third and fourth cleansing was statistically lower than during the first and second ($p = 0.039$). Malmros et al. suggest that this might have resulted from psychological conditioning, a different absorption rate for the anesthetics or reduced wound hyperalgesia (possibly due to anti-inflammatory effects of the local anesthetics). Cleansing was considered satisfactory in all patients, and the investigators concluded that the use of EMLA cream in this study provided sufficient pain control in 95% of treatments.

Local reactions included a burning sensation (four patients), itching (one patient), pallor (three patients) and redness (two patients).

Study 2

Wanger et al. [7] investigated the efficacy of EMLA during frequent and repeated use for leg ulcer debridement. Thirty patients with ulcers of arterial, venous or vasculitic origin received EMLA topical anesthesia for surgical debridement taking place either three times a week for 2 weeks or once a week for 2 months. No significant differences in pain reduction were noted over the course of the repeated treatments and the authors concluded that EMLA provided, in the majority of patients studied, sufficient anesthesia to allow for adequate debridement. Side effects (edema, itching or burning) were mild and did not increase on repeated application. Bacterial flora did not show any clinically important change during the course of the study, and no signs of clinical infection were observed in the skin surrounding the ulcers.

Study 3

The issue of repeating topical analgesia with EMLA prior to mechanical debridement of leg ulcers was also addressed by Hansson and co-workers [8]. Forty-three patients with venous leg ulcers were assessed in an open, randomized, parallel-group study. EMLA was applied as a thick cream 30 minutes prior to eight serial surgical debridements in 22 patients, while the control group (21 patients) received no topical cream prior to the debridement. Pain was assessed by the patient using a VAS. The EMLA group experienced significantly less pain during and after the debridement, and the analgesic effect remained unchanged with each successive treatment. No serious adverse reactions were noted, and the healing rate was similar in both groups. The bacterial flora was as expected in venous ulcers at the start and finish of the study in both groups. No signs of clinical infection were observed in the skin surrounding the ulcer during the 2-month trial.

III. CONCLUSIONS

Review of the literature suggests that EMLA sterile cream produces
safe and effective topical analgesia when used in the debridement of
leg ulcers of vascular origin. To be effective, it appears that an adequate
amount of cream must be applied, preferably under occlusion, between
30 and 60 minutes prior to the surgical procedure. EMLA sterile cream
does not appear to increase the risk of infection. Plasma concentrations
of lidocaine and prilocaine were considerably lower than those associated with toxicity, although it should be kept in mind that the absorption
of these two topical anesthetics will increase if used on ulcers of
increasing size. No major adverse effects have been reported during
use of EMLA for the relief of pain associated with ulcer debridement.
Common side effects, which we consider minor, are described as slight
or moderate burning, local redness and pallor. These effects occur in
only a small proportion of patients.

Used appropriately, this unique topical anesthetic cream should
enhance the ability of physicians to surgically debride leg ulcers of
vascular origin, thus reducing the time needed for the healing of such
ulcers.

REFERENCES

1. Callam MJ: Chronic ulceration of the leg. Br Med J 1987: 294; 1389-1391.

2. Anderson E, Hansson C, Swan Beek G: Leg and foot ulcers. An epi-
    demiological survey. Acta Derm Venereol (Stockh) 1984; 64: 227-232.

3. Larsson B Stymne, Rotstein A, Widman M: Clinical Dermatology in
    the Year 2000, meeting, London, May 1990, pp 22-25.

4. Enander-Malmros E, Nilsen T, Lillieborg S: Plasma concentrations and
    analgesic effect of EMLA (Lidocaine/Prilocaine) cream for the cleans-
    ing of leg ulcers. Acta Derm Venereol (Stockh) 1990; 70: 227-230.

5. Holm J, Andren B, Grafford K: Pain control in the surgical debridement
    of leg ulcers by the use of a topical lidocaine/prilocaine cream, EMLA.
    Acta Derm Venereol (Stockh) 1990; 70: 132-136.

6. Rosenthal D, Murphy F, Gottschalk R et al.: A double blind placebo
    controlled study of lidocaine/prilocaine cream (EMLA®) used as a

topical analgesic for mechanical debridement of leg ulcers. Can Med Assoc J. Submitted October 1993.

7. Wanger L, Eriksson C, Karlsson A: Analgesic effect and local reactions of repeated application of EMLA (lidocaine/prilocaine) cream for the cleansing of leg ulcers (abstr). Clinical Dermatology in the Year 2000, meeting, London, May 1990.

8. Hansson C, Holm J, Lillieborg S, Syren A: Repeated treatment with lidocaine/prilocaine cream (EMLA) as a topical anaesthetic for the cleansing of venous leg ulcers: A controlled study. Acta Derm Venereol (Stockh) 1993; 73: 231-233.

12

Use of EMLA Cream in Hemodialysis Patients

Izhar ul Qamar

University of Chicago
Chicago, Illinois

I. INTRODUCTION

Hemodialysis patients suffer repeated pain associated with the procedures of cannulation and dialysis that are needed to maintain their homeostasis. Several recent studies have investigated the use of EMLA® cream to provide analgesia for such patients during insertion of the large-gauge needles required for dialysis. This chapter discusses the epidemiology, nature and problems associated with end-stage renal failure, and reviews evidence on the efficacy of EMLA cream in improving the quality of life of these patients.

Table 1 Epidemiology of End-Stage Renal Failure

Country [Ref.]	Patients on renal replacement therapy		Frequency of end-stage renal failure	Incidence of new cases per year
	1990	1991	(No. patients per million population)	
Europe [a]				
Total [1]	152,658	168,927	24.5	48 (1991)
Pediatric [2]	8,894		19.5	2.8
U.S. [3]	160,000 (1989)			
Canada [4]				45 (1981)
				80 (1990)

[a] Data from 36 countries.

II. END-STAGE RENAL DISEASE

Renal failure, defined as a decrease in the renal function to a level insufficient to maintain homeostasis, can be of acute or chronic onset. Various stages of renal disease can occur, with end-stage renal disease (ESRD) being characterized by residual renal function varying between 2% and 20% of the normal. Prior to the introduction of various renal replacement therapies, such as hemodialysis, peritoneal dialysis and renal transplantation, end-stage renal failure was universally fatal as recent as 40 years ago.

Epidemiological data for end-stage renal failure in Europe, Canada and the United States are given in Table 1. The number of patients receiving treatment appears to be increasing, and in Europe 33,032 new patients were accepted for treatment of end-stage renal failure during 1991.

The technique of extracorporeal dialysis of blood as a means of sustaining life in patients with otherwise fatal acute renal failure was developed over a number of years [5–7]. With the introduction of the Quinton Scribner shunt in 1960 [8], allowing repeated access to blood vessels, hemodialysis became possible as a renal replacement therapy for ESRD.

The process of hemodialysis consists of extracorporeal circulation of a patient's blood through a dialyser, whereby the toxic waste products are removed and the blood returned to the patient. Successful hemodialysis as maintenance therapy in ESRD depends upon availability of a stable vascular access. This may be achieved through an external arteriovenous shunt [8], an internal arteriovenous fistula [9] or central venous catheters; an internal arteriovenous fistula in the lower forearm is currently the most common type of vascular access.

Chronic hemodialysis involves cannulation of the arteriovenous fistula with a wide-bore needle (15 to 18 gauge). This cannulation procedure, which can be painful, has to be repeated two to three times a week. Hemodialysis patients, especially children, requiring cannulation of arteriovenous fistula may have adverse psychological effects as a result of the pain and discomfort caused by the procedure. Moreover, previous and cumulative painful experiences induce a high level of anxiety at each subsequent procedure. Psychological and emotional adjustment to the treatment of chronic renal failure can be difficult [10–12]. For example, repeated and potentially painful dialysis sessions, rigid dialysis schedules and dietary restrictions all contribute to the strain on such patients. Social and psychological factors have a major influence on their quality of life [13].

The objective of management of ESRD should include improving the quality of patient's life. Pain from repeated venipuncture of the arteriovenous fistula for hemodialysis could be emotionally traumatic, especially in children, and could add to the various other stresses to which a patient with ESRD is exposed. It would therefore seem desirable to avoid the pain of cannulation of arteriovenous fistulas during hemodialysis sessions as one of the measures to improve quality of life for these patients.

III. EMLA CREAM IN HEMODIALYSIS PATIENTS

Given the effectiveness of EMLA cream in preventing pain of venipuncture (Chapter 3), it appears most appropriate to use it for that purpose in hemodialysis patients who undergo cannulation of the arteriovenous fistula two to three times a week. Several long-term studies investigating the use of EMLA cream in hemodialysis patients have been reported.

A. Study 1

In a randomized double-blind, placebo-controlled, cross-over study, Watson et al. [14] compared the anaesthetic effect of EMLA cream to that of topical placebo or lidocaine injections in arteriovenous fistula cannulation. Twenty-six hemodialysis patients (19 male and seven female), aged between 19 and 70 years, were recruited into the study. Prior to enrollment, all patients regularly used intradermal injections of lidocaine to provide local anaesthesia during cannulation. The patient's usual technique of lidocaine injection was assessed on day 1 of the study, followed by random assignment of EMLA or placebo cream application during the second and third sessions of hemodialysis. The creams were applied in a thick layer under an occlusive dressing at least 60 minutes prior to the fistula cannulation. The pain of cannulation was assessed on a visual analog scale (VAS) and a 4-point verbal rating scale.

Eighteen patients (70%) in the placebo group required supplementary injections of lidocaine compared to 3 (11%) in the EMLA group ($p < 0.001$). There was a significant decrease in pain associated with cannulation when EMLA cream was used compared to that experienced with placebo as assessed by both the VAS and verbal rating scale. The pain with EMLA cream was also less when compared to the lidocaine injection results, being statistically significant on the VAS only. Many of the patients expressed a strong preference for EMLA cream over lidocaine injection, because they had experienced discomfort and apprehension during infiltration of the latter.

With the exception of one patient who developed severe itching and rash 10 hours after application of EMLA cream, local skin reactions, mainly skin blanching, were reported as being mild and transient.

B. Study 2

Andersen et al. [15] studied the analgesic effects of EMLA cream used over a median period of 5 months in 22 hemodialysis patients (aged 12 to 67 years), all of whom had experienced pain and discomfort during routine cannulation of the arteriovenous fistula prior to the study. The degree of pain experienced without analgesia was assessed at the time of entry into the study, by both an observing nurse and the patient, using a 3-point verbal scale. A thick layer of EMLA cream (2.5 g) was applied under occlusion (Tegaderm®) for at least 60 minutes prior to the cannulation procedure. A total of 2227 applications of EMLA cream were recorded in the 22 patients; 13 patients completed the study.

A verbal rating of "no pain" was reported in 87% of the cannulations, with moderate pain in 10% and severe pain in 1.5% after EMLA cream application. Pruritus and redness were reported as the most common local reactions, with one patient discontinuing treatment due to these reactions.

C. Study 3

Wehle et al. [16] reported on repeated long-term use of EMLA cream over a period of 1 to 1.5 years (300 to 312 applications of EMLA cream), for alleviation of pain of cannulation in 31 hemodialysis patients aged between 48 and 75 years (median 66 years). Seventeen patients completed the study. A thick layer (2.5 g) of 5% EMLA cream was applied under occlusive dressing for a median period of 95 minutes (SD ± 26.5). Two fistula needles (15 and 18 gauge) were used for cannulation of the arteriovenous fistula. The analgesic effect of EMLA was compared with a placebo cream in a double-blind randomized fashion on a regular basis. Pain experienced during cannulation was assessed by the patient using a VAS.

EMLA cream was found to alleviate pain of cannulation significantly when compared to the placebo. No significant change in perception of pain was noticed with chronic use of EMLA cream, suggesting lack of tolerance. The analgesic effects were found to be equal for both the venous and the arterial sites of the arteriovenous fistula. The majority (66%) of applications were reported without any local skin reactions. Local pallor was the most frequently observed reaction, with local redness being the second most common. Itching, burning sensation and edema were reported as occasional, as were spongy or rough skin and temporary eczematous skin irritation.

IV. CONCLUSION

The studies mentioned above prove the efficacy of both short- and long-term use of EMLA cream in alleviating the pain associated with cannulation of arteriovenous fistula in hemodialysis patients. No significant adverse effects were associated with repeated applications of the cream.

Young pediatric patients are most susceptible to the harmful emotional and psychological effects of the pain and discomfort associated with arteriovenous fistula cannulation. Studies conducted to date have involved mainly adult patients with some older children; therefore further studies on the safety and efficacy of EMLA cream for this indication in a pediatric population are urgently needed.

ESRD patients are already burdened with stresses associated with their disease. The cost of EMLA cream application should be weighed against the benefits of avoidance of repeated emotional trauma and discomfort with its consequent harmful long-term psychological effects. This pain-prevention measure has the potential of substantially improving the quality of life of patients during hemodialysis.

REFERENCES

1. Raine AEG, Margreiter R, Brunner FP et al.: Report on management of renal failure in Europe, XXII, 1991. Nephrol Dial Transplant 1992; Suppl 2: 7-35.
2. Ehrich JHH, Loirat C, Brunner FP et al.: Report on management of renal failure in children in Europe, XXII, 1991. Nephrol Dial Transplant 1992; Suppl 2: 36-48.
3. U.S. Renal Data System: USRDS 1991 annual data report. Am J Kidney Dis 1991; 5 (Suppl 2): 1-27.

4. Fenton SSA: All patients and facilities. In: Canadian Organ Replacement Register 1990 Report. Hospital Medical Records Institute, Don Mills, Ontario.

5. Munro AC: Thomas Graham (1805-1869). Phil J (Glasgow) 1971; 8: 30.

6. Abel JJ, Rowntree LG, Turner BB: On the removal of diffusible substances from circulating blood by means of dialysis. Trans Assoc Am Phys 1913; 28: 51.

7. Kolff WJ: First clinical experience with the artificial kidney. Ann Intern Med 1965; 62: 608.

8. Quinton WE, Dillard D, Scribner BH: Cannulation of blood vessels for prolonged hemodialysis. Trans Am Soc Artif Intern Organs 1960; 6: 104-113.

9. Brescia MJ, Cimino JE, Appel K, Hurwich BJ: Chronic hemodialysis using venipuncture and a surgically created arterio venous fistula. N Engl J Med 1966; 275: 1089-1092.

10. Blodgett CJ: A selected review of the literature of adjustment to hemodialysis. Int J Psychiatry Med 1981-82; 11: 97-124.

11. Blodgett CJ: The process of adjustment in chronic renal failure and hemodialysis. Disserta Abstr Int 1983; 44: 905B.

12. Hilbert GA: An investigation of the relationship between social support and compliance of hemodialysis patients. Am Nephrol Nurs Assoc J 1985; 12: 133-136.

13. Devins GM, Binik YM, Hollomby DJ et al.: Helplessness and depression in end-stage renal disease. J Abnorm Psychol 1981; 90: 531-545.

14. Watson AR, Szymkiw P, Morgan AG: Topical anaesthesia for fistula cannulation in hemodialysis patients. Nephrol Dial Transplant 1988; 3:800-802.

15. Andersen C, Danielson K, Ladefoged J: EMLA cream for pain prevention in hemodialysis patients. Dialysis Transplantation 1989; 18: 684-685.

16. Wehle B, Bjornstrom M, Cedgard M, et al. Repeated application of EMLA cream 5% for the alleviation of cannulation pain in hemodialysis. Scand J Urol Nephrol 1989; 23: 299-302.

13

The Emerging Role of EMLA Cream in Lithotripsy

Kathleen Shilalukey

University of Zambia
Lusaka, Zambia

I. INTRODUCTION

Urolithiasis, or stone (calculi) formation in the urinary tract, occurs when the balance between solute excretion and water conservation in the kidney is disturbed by factors such as diet, exercise and excessive solute load [1]. Countries with a high annual stone frequency include the United Kingdom, Scandinavia and the United States, the last having an annual incidence of more than one stone per 1000 population [2].

Coates first investigated the potential for ultrasonic destruction of human calculi in the 1940s. By 1950, biliary calculi could be fragmented [3], and fragmentation of urinary calculi was possible by

1955; invasive methods were used during these early procedures. During the late 1970s and early 1980s, percutaneous procedures became popular for disintegration of both small and large stones. Extracorporeal shock-wave lithotripsy (ESWL) was introduced in the mid-1980s, and today this technique represents the most common therapy for renal calculi [4].

ESWL, carried out as first described with instruments such as the Dornier HM3 lithotriptor, was a painful process that required regional or general anesthesia [5]. The ultrasonic energy range used during early work with such instruments was 18 to 24 kV. However, modifications to the lithotriptor instruments (e.g. reflector geometry and generator capacitance) and/or methods used [4] have allowed lithotripsy to be performed at lower energies (e.g. 14 to 16 kV) without such anesthesia. Provision of premedication together with local anesthesia of the skin at the point of entry of the shock waves is generally sufficient to allow patients to tolerate the procedure.

The stone burden directly affects the morbidity associated with ESWL, and is inversely related to the success of the procedure [6]. Morbidity is also higher with staghorn calculi and in cases of multiple nephrostomies, retrograde uretroscopy and ureteral obstruction by a column of fragments ("steinstrasse"). Pain experienced during extracorporeal shock wave lithotripsy arises from two sources: a visceral or deep pain within the body and pain felt at the body surface during impact of the shock waves [7].

This chapter focuses on the efficacy of EMLA® cream in alleviating the pain experienced in the skin during urological procedures such as lithotripsy.

II. THE USE OF EMLA CREAM IN ESWL

A randomized, double-blind, placebo-controlled trial was conducted by Bierkens et al. [8] to determine the therapeutic efficacy of EMLA cream during ESWL for urinary calculi. A total of 83 patients were enrolled; EMLA or placebo cream was applied to the skin (100 cm^2) at the site of the shock-head coupling. Of the 40 patients treated with

EMLA cream, 12 (30%) required supplementary analgesia with i.v. fentanyl citrate, compared to 23 (53%) of the 43 placebo-treated patients. Bierkens et al. noted that in their general population of patients treated with a Siemens Lithostar lithotriptor, 51% normally required i.v. analgesia. Although the difference between EMLA and placebo found during the trial was not statistically significant, the EMLA cream was observed to decrease pain during ESWL; hence the authors considered it useful for patients in whom i.v. analgesia is contraindicated [16].

Tiselius [9] carried out a randomized, double-blind, placebo-controlled trial in a total of 199 patients undergoing ESWL with an unmodified Dornier HM3 lithotriptor. ESWL was started at a low kilovoltage level and increased as necessary. All patients received premedication with meperidine HCl and diazepam; 99 patients were randomized to EMLA cream (application time at least 60 minutes) and 100 patients received placebo. The requirement for additional analgesic sedation at each voltage, together with pain scores (6-point scale) and overall treatment acceptability (4-point scale), was noted in each group.

Results from this study [9] are shown in Table 1. At 14 kV, additional analgesia was required in significantly more patients in the placebo group than in the EMLA group ($p < 0.05$). This difference varied according to the stone position, and was most pronounced in a subgroup of patients with stones in the upper calices. It was noted that, while the number of women who received additional analgesia was equal for the placebo and EMLA groups, the number of men in the placebo group who required additional analgesia was significantly greater than in the EMLA group.

The authors concluded that EMLA cream provided clinically significant improvements in the pain experienced during ESWL, and could be used to reduce the dose of analgesic and sedative drugs administered during the procedure.

Pettersson et al. [4] conducted a study designed to investigate the efficacy and acceptability of a modified ESWL procedure, using an unmodified Dornier HM3 lithotriptor (energy range 14 to 16 kV), in 210 patients given premedication (pethidine and diazepam) and

Table 1 Results from Tiselius's Study of 199 Patients Undergoing ESWL

Treatment	EMLA group	Placebo group
No. of patients	99	100
No. of patients not requiring additional analgesia:		
14 kV	73	58
19 kV	50	0
ESWL completed without additional analgesia	50%	39%
Percentage of patients *requiring* additional analgesia at 14 kV for:		
Stones in upper calices	22%	79%
Men/women	14%/33%	88%/67%
Stones in middle calices	37%	57%
Stones in lower calices	25%	39%
Pelvic stones	23%	23%
Proximal ureteral stones	30%	40%
Mid-ureteral stones	0%	29%
All stones		
No. of men	13	29
No. of women	13	13
All stones, overall	26%	42%
Pain scores	2.40 ± 0.91	2.64 ± 1.08
Acceptability assessment	2.95 ± 0.58	3.18 ± 1.27
No. of patients with supplementary meperidine dose:		
≤ 25 mg	32	31
> 25 mg	18	31

Source: Ref. 9.

EMLA analgesia over the site of shock-wave entry. Results were compared to those previously obtained using the original procedure, with a generator voltage of 18 to 23 kV in patients under anesthesia. Using the modified method, over 90% of patients reported the pain experienced during ESWL to be acceptable and of moderate intensity or less; only 3% found the treatment unpleasant. The final therapeutic result was the same for both the modified and the unmodified method, although the modified method required a greater number of treatments for large or ureteral stones.

De Lichtenberg et al. compared the anesthetic efficacy of EMLA cream with that of lidocaine infiltration in a study of 91 patients undergoing ESWL (16 to 18 kV energy) [10]. In 46 patients, EMLA cream (30 g) was applied over the kidney 90 minutes before commencing ESWL. Lidocaine with adrenaline (20 ml, 1% solution) was administered by subcutaneous infiltration to the remaining 45 patients. The two groups were well matched for demographic details and ESWL treatment required. All patients received morphine immediately prior to ESWL. The researchers found no significant difference between the two groups in the median pain score or in the amount of supplementary analgesics required, and concluded that, if correctly applied, EMLA cream could be recommended for ESWL.

A placebo-controlled, randomized, double-blind study was conducted by Monk et al. [11] in 58 patients undergoing lithotripsy with the Dormer HM3 lithotriptor. EMLA cream (30 patients) or placebo (28 patients) was applied over the kidney (30 g cream over 200 cm^2, 90-minute application time). All patients received midazolam premedication. Test shocks were given at 10, 12, 15, 18 and 20 kV to determine the relationship between pain intensity and shock energy; shocks were discontinued if the patient complained of severe pain or if their visual analog score (scale of 0 to 100) was greater than 70. Pain scores were significantly lower in patients treated with EMLA cream for test shocks at 15, 18 and 20 kV. This study [11] also detected a significant difference in the efficacy of EMLA cream between men and women patients, with higher efficacy found in men.

III. DISCUSSION

When ESWL was first introduced, general or epidural anesthesia were recommended. However, experience with the use of local anesthetics in lithotripsy has increased, and in some centers general anesthesia is now used in only 6 to 10% of patients [12]. Approximately 75% of patients in a study reported by Lingeman et al. [12] were willing to repeat ESWL treatment under local anesthesia. Following lithotripsy with local anesthesia, stone-free success rates are 74 to 99% [13,14], with acceptable retreatment rates of about 35% being reported [14].

Local anesthesia offers many advantages over general or epidural anesthesia for lithotripsy, both for the patient and for the physicians carrying out the procedure. Patients do not suffer the side effects of nausea, vomiting, etc., that are common with general anesthesia, and recover from local anesthetics more quickly. Remote monitoring of vital signs and positioning of the patient in the lithotripsy immersion tank can be difficult for the anesthetist and physicians when the patient is unconscious after treatment with general anesthesia. Conversely, patients treated with local anesthetics who are conscious can be asked to cooperate during the operation, if necessary [15].

The above studies show that, in premedicated patients, the efficacy of EMLA cream is significantly better than placebo, and equal to that provided by local infiltration of lidocaine. Advantages of EMLA cream include the easy and pain-free administration of the cream, and the absence of any bleeding from needle punctures, which can pose a viral-infection risk to medical workers.

Potential drawbacks of EMLA cream are the prolonged application time required (60 to 90 minutes) and difficulty in defining in advance the required area of application over the site of entry of shock waves. Theoretical problems such as risk of cannular infection (if non-sterile cream were to be used) or systemic absorption of lidocaine and prilocaine have not been encountered in clinical practice. Although none of the above studies investigated serum levels of local anesthetics following EMLA cream application in lithotripsy, available kinetic data suggest that serum concentrations do not reach clinically relevant levels (see Chapters 2 and 11). Further studies may be required to verify the gender-related differences observed for EMLA cream efficacy in one study during lithotripsy.

IV. CONCLUSION

EMLA cream appears to be a viable and effective form of anesthesia-analgesia in lithotripsy. EMLA cream local anesthesia has advantages over general anesthesia in that the patient is concious during the operation, and, in contrast to infiltration local anesthetics, administration of the cream is pain-free.

REFERENCES

1. Smith LJ: The medical aspects of urolithiasis: an overview. J Urol 1988; 141: 707.
2. Straffon RA, Higgins CC: Urolithiasis. In: Urology. Campbell MR, Harrison JH, eds. WB Saunders, Philadelphia, 1970; pp 687-757.
3. Motola JA, Smith AD: Therapeutic options for the management of upper tract calculi. Urol Clin North Am 1990; 17(1): 191-205.
4. Pettersson B, Tiselius HG, Andersson A, Eriksson I: Evaluation of extracorporeal shock wave lithotripsy without anesthesia using a Dornier HM3 lithotriptor without technical modifications. J Urol 1989; 142: 1189-1192.
5. Jocham D, Chaussy C, Schmiedt E: Extracorporeal shock wave lithotripsy. Urol Internat 1986; 41: 357-368.
6. Lingeman JE, Newman DM, Mertz JHO: Extracorporeal shock wave lithotripsy: The Methodist Hospital of Indiana experience. J Urol 1986; 135: 1134.
7. Malhotra V, Long CW, Meister MJ: Intercostal blocks with local infiltration anesthesia for extracorporeal shock wave lithotripsy. Anesth Analg 1987; 66: 85-88.
8. Bierkens FA, Maes MR, Hendriky MJ, Erdos AF, de Vries JDM, Debruyne FMJ: The use of local anesthesia in second generation extracorporeal shock wave lithotripsy: eutectic mixture of local anesthetics. J Urol 1991; 146: 287-289.
9. Tiselius HG: Cutaneous anaesthesia with lidocaine-prilocaine cream: A useful adjunct during shock wave lithotripsy with analgesic sedation. J Urol 1993; 149: 8-11.
10. De Lichtenberg MH, Misokoniak J, Mogensen P, Andersen JT: Local anesthesia for extracorporeal shock wave lithotripsy. A study comparing eutectic mixture of local anesthetic cream and lidocaine infiltration. J Urol 1992; 147: 96-97
11. Monk TG, Ding Y, White PF: Analgesic efficacy of EMLA during outpatient shock wave lithotripsy. Anesth Analg 1992; 74: S213.
12. Lingeman JE, Shirrek WL, Newman DM, Mosbaugh PG, Steele RE, Woods JR: Management of upper ureteral calculi with extracorporeal shock wave lithotripsy. J Urol 1987; 138: 720-723.

13. Holden D , Rao PN: Ureteral stones: the result of primary in situ extracorporeal shock wave lithoptripsy. J Urol 1989; 142: 37-39.
14. Tiselius H-G: Anaesthesia-free in situ extracorporeal shock wave lithotripsy of ureteral stones. J Urol 1991; 146: 8-12.
15. Malhotra V, Long CW, Meister MJ: Intercostal blocks with local infiltration anesthesia for extracorporeal shock wave lithotripsy. Anesth Analg 1987; 66: 85-88.

14

Use of EMLA Cream in Otolaryngology

Doreen Matsui

Children's Hospital of Western Ontario
London, Ontario, Canada

Matitiahu Berkovitch

Assaf Harofe Hospital
Tzrifim, Israel

I. INTRODUCTION

In England and Wales, otitis media with effusion is the most common indication for childhood surgery [1]. In the United States, an estimated 1 million children undergo myringotomy and tympanostomy tube insertion every year, this procedure being the most common minor surgical operation performed under general anesthesia [2].

For many years otologists have searched for an alternative to general anesthesia, in particular a safe and effective method of producing local anesthesia of the external meatus and tympanic membrane. A variety of methods have been used with varying degrees of success and adverse effects. Local anesthetic agents such as topical cocaine and lidocaine are rapidly absorbed by mucosal surfaces; however, they do not readily penetrate normal epidermis, including the external surface of the tympanic membrane and meatal skin [3].

Attempts have been made to increase the effectiveness of local anesthetics by the application of local irritants, such as phenol, which increase the surface vascularity and thereby facilitate transfer of the local anesthetic [4]. In the past, otologists used a solution of 5% sodium bicarbonate and glycerine to macerate the keratin layer of the tympanic membrane followed by a mixture of alcohol and cocaine as an anesthetic. A mixture known as Bonain's solution, composed of phenol, menthol and cocaine (with or without adrenaline), has also been employed to destroy the superficial layers of the tympanic membrane. Unfortunately the use of these necrotizing solutions is fraught with problems such as systemic absorption and toxicity, drum perforation, damage to the vestibulocochlear apparatus and facial palsy [3].

Local infiltration of the meatus offers an effective alternative, but the pain of the injection is a major drawback. In addition, it may be difficult to inject the anterior wall of the ear canal close enough to the annulus to adequately anesthetize this part of the tympanic membrane [3]. Iontophoresis has been employed to improve the passage of the local anesthetic across the epithelial barrier of the tympanic membrane. This technique involves the use of a low-amperage direct current from a positive electrode to drive positive ions of the agent through the tympanic membrane, which is the path of least resistance [5]. Disadvantages of this method are that it is cumbersome and time-consuming, and does not provide effective anesthesia of the skin of the external canal [3].

Given the lack of a satisfactory method of local anesthesia for otolaryngological procedures, and the risks and costs of general anesthesia, there is much interest in new possibilities, in particular those that are practical in an outpatient setting. EMLA® cream has been shown to reduce the pain of venipuncture [6,7], and its application has been extended to the field of otolaryngology with impressive results.

II. CLINICAL STUDIES

The most widespread study of EMLA cream in this therapeutic area has involved anesthesia of the tympanic membrane, in particular, for myringotomy and ventilation tube insertion procedures. In most cases, EMLA cream is instilled into the external auditory canal covering the tympanic membrane, using a syringe and cannula under the direct vision of a microscope. The cream is left in situ for a designated period of time (reports vary from 15 minutes to 3 hours) and then removed. Several clinical trials comparing EMLA cream to no treatment, placebo cream or standard anesthesia such as cocaine or lidocaine (spray or infiltration) have been reported. Most of the trials have been conducted in adults, with pain being scored using a visual analog scale (VAS).

In a double-blind trial [3], 15 patients, aged 15 to 67 years, underwent bilateral electrocochleography with EMLA cream applied to one ear and placebo (hand cream) to the other. In all cases the EMLA-treated ear was described as being more comfortable. No change in pure-tone audiometry was demonstrated and no tinnitus or vertigo was reported. Thirty patients subsequently underwent various procedures, including electrocochleography, myringotomy and grommet insertion, with successful results using EMLA cream.

In another double-blind study [8], 20 adult patients were randomly allocated to receive either EMLA or placebo cream. A further 10 patients received prilocaine injections. Myringotomy, aspiration of effusion and grommet insertion were performed. Both EMLA cream and injected prilocaine were equally effective in anesthetizing the tympanic membrane, and were significantly better than placebo. However, the pain associated with the injection of the prilocaine was rated as being similar to that experienced with grommet insertion without anesthesia, while the insertion of EMLA cream was relatively painless.

Whittett et al. [9] compared the anesthesia achieved using EMLA cream with that provided by the more traditional 5% cocaine solution in a single-blind controlled trial involving 49 patients, aged 16 to 79 years. The anesthetic was introduced into the ear, and myringotomy (followed in some cases by fluid aspiration and grommet insertion) was undertaken. For all three procedures, significantly less discomfort was noted with the use of EMLA cream than with cocaine. In addition, three patients in the cocaine group suffered vertigo and nystagmus, a complication not seen in the EMLA group.

Another study [10] involved 42 voluntary subjects, aged 21 to 36 years, who received EMLA cream in one ear and either Bonain's solution or 10% lidocaine spray (due to side effects encountered with the Bonain's solution) in the other ear. Pain and sense of touch experienced by the tympanic membrane and posterior ear canal skin were tested using a cotton-tipped wire. Full anesthesia was attained with EMLA cream significantly more often than with lidocaine and almost significantly more often than with Bonain's solution. Most individuals judged the EMLA-treated ear to be better anesthetized. Undesired side effects, including two tympanic membrane perforations, appeared in most of the ears anesthetized with Bonain's solution.

In a second phase of this study [10], myringotomy, tympanostomy tube insertion or other minor surgical operations were performed under EMLA anesthesia in 127 ears. The procedures were rated as painless in 83 ears, unpleasant in 36, and painful in eight. The authors recommend that Bonain's solution should be replaced by EMLA cream or a corresponding agent for local anesthesia of the tympanic membrane.

Sirimanna et al. [5] compared EMLA cream to iontophoresis in a total of 35 patients undergoing myringotomy and grommet insertion with fluid aspiration if necessary. No significant difference in pain scores was noted between the EMLA ($n = 15$) and the iontophoresis ($n = 20$) treatment groups. EMLA cream appeared to provide better anesthesia of the skin of the external canal and was considered to be a more efficient technique with regard to preparation time.

In a preliminary study, Bingham et al. [11] utilized EMLA cream in eight patients undergoing various minor otological procedures; all patients denied sensing pain during their operation. EMLA cream was then used in another 29 adult patients (37 tympanic membranes) undergoing myringotomy with or without ventilation tube insertion [12]. All patients tolerated the operative procedure well, and those with previous experience of anesthetic techniques expressed a preference for EMLA cream. The patients did not complain of vertigo or tinnitus, and no evidence of alteration in sensorineural thresholds was demonstrated by pure-tone audiometry.

Hickey et al. [4] reported a technique, carried out under EMLA anesthesia, for myringotomy and suctioning of middle-ear effusion, followed by ventilation-tube insertion if required. This procedure could be performed without difficulty in patients older than 12 years of age and has been used in children as young as 5 years old.

In this study [4], myringotomy, and in some cases ventilation-tube insertion, was undertaken using EMLA cream in 109 children, aged 3 to 12 years, with the procedure failing in only seven (6.8%). The failures tended to occur in younger children and in most cases at the time of myringotomy. Of note, in this study the EMLA cream was applied to the ear canal for 3 hours. The authors emphasized that a penetration time of at least 2 hours is required for adequate anesthesia, since the only acceptable pain level in the paediatric age group is nil. Complications occurred in two children: one patient with an obstructed tube and the other a premature extrusion of the tube. Ninety-two of the 94 children who had ventilation tubes inserted had normal post-operative audiograms. In the remaining two children, there were other possible explanations for abnormal audiograms [13].

Kaddour [14] carried out fat-graft myringoplasty as day care surgery in 11 patients (aged 15 to 51 years), using EMLA anesthesia. All patients had dry central perforations covering 30% or less of the tympanic membrane. The fat graft was harvested under lidocaine infiltration anesthesia and the grafting carried out following application of EMLA cream to the tympanic membrane and ear canal for 1 hour. On a 4-point verbal rating scale, patients assessed the procedure as painless or slightly uncomfortable. A 3-month follow-up in 10 patients showed that eight perforations were completely closed. The author concluded that the outpatient operation was safe, reliable and cost-effective.

Although most of the published studies describing the use of EMLA cream in otolaryngology pertain to anesthesia of the tympanic membrane for myringotomy and tympanostomy tube insertion, EMLA cream has been tried in other settings in this field. For example, using EMLA cream as a topical analgesic, Premachandra [15] treated two patients with furuncles of the external auditory meatus and three patients with painful otitis externa. A significant reduction in pain was noted. EMLA cream also facilitated thorough cleaning of the ear canal of infected debris prior to application of topical antibiotics [15].

Twelve patients, aged 16 to 30 years, had simple fractures of their nasal bones reduced without pain after application of EMLA cream to a designated area of skin covering the nose and of 5% cocaine solution to the nasal mucosa [16]. Successful manipulation with good cosmetic result was carried out in all patients except one, in whom the failure was attributed to a previous fracture.

III. PRECLINICAL OTOTOXICITY STUDIES

Instillation of EMLA cream into the middle ear of guinea pigs resulted in severe morphological damage to localized areas of the organ of Corti, while only minor changes occurred in the middle ear. Vestibular symptoms were noted, as were reversible effects on hearing thresholds and latencies. When EMLA cream was introduced into the external auditory canal with an intact tympanic membrane, no morphological changes were detected in either the middle or inner ear [17]. Anniko et al. [18] instilled EMLA cream into the round window niche of rats and found severe morphological degeneration in the basal part of the cochlea. Functional impairment was demonstrated by auditory brain-stem recordings. EMLA cream has also been applied to the tympanic membrane of rats and guinea pigs with few if any signs of epithelial reaction and no effect on connective tissue [19]. Varied morphological and functional changes have also been noted with other agents that have been used to anesthetize the ear [18,19].

Although these animal studies raise concerns regarding the oto-toxic potential of EMLA cream, major complications have not been encountered when it has been used for anesthesia for otological procedures. Use of EMLA cream is not recommended in the presence of a perforated tympanic membrane because systemic absorption of its constituent local anesthetic agents will be increased if it comes in direct contact with the middle ear mucosa [5], and because of the theoretical risk of contaminating the round or oval windows [3]. Prior to the surgical procedure, all cream should be removed from the meatus and tympanic membrane [3]. If EMLA cream is used properly for myringotomy and ventilation-tube-insertion procedures, inner ear damage should be only a remote theoretical risk [12].

IV. CONCLUSION

Although not recommended in the prescribing information, a large body of work to date suggests that EMLA cream is a promising alternative to the less than satisfactory methods of anesthesia available to the otolaryngologist today.

REFERENCES

1. Black N: Surgery for glue ear: a modern epidemic. Lancet 1984; i: 835-837.
2. Bluestone C: Otitis media in children: to treat or not to treat? N Engl J Med 1982; 306: 1399-1404.
3. Timms MS, O'Malley S, Keith AO: Experience with a new topical anaesthetic in otolaryngology. Clin Otolaryngol 1988; 13: 485-490.
4. Hickey SA, Buckley JG, Fitzgerald O'Conner AF: Ventilation tube insertion under local anesthesia. Am J Otolaryngol 1991; 12: 142-143.
5. Sirmanna KS, Madden GJ, Miles S: Anaesthesia of the tympanic membrane: comparison of EMLA cream and iontophoresis. J Laryngol Otol 1990; 104: 195-196.
6. Hallen B, Carlsson P, Uppfeldt A: Clinical study of a lignocaine-prilocaine cream to relieve the pain of venepuncture. Br J Anaesth 1985; 57: 326-328.
7. Robieux I, Kumar R, Radhakrishnan S, Koren G: Assessing pain and analgesia with a lidocaine-prilocaine emulsion in infants and toddlers during venipuncture. J Pediat 1991; 118: 971-973.
8. Roberts C, Carlin WV: A comparison of topical EMLA cream and prilocaine injection for anaesthesia of the tympanic membrane in adults. Acta Otolaryngol (Stockh) 1989; 108: 431-433.
9. Whittet HB, Williams HO, Wright A: An evaluation of topical anaesthesia for myringotomy. Clin Otolaryngol 1988; 13: 481-484.
10. Luotonen J, Laitakari K, Karjalainen H, Jokinen K: EMLA in local anaesthesia of the tympanic membrane. Acta Otolaryngol (Stockh) Suppl 1992; 492: 63-67.

11. Bingham B, Hawthorne M: The use of anaesthetic EMLA cream in minor otological surgery. J Laryngol Otol 1988; 102: 517.

12. Bingham B, Hawke M, Halik J: The safety and efficacy of EMLA cream topical anesthesia for myringotomy and ventilation tube insertion. J Otolaryngol 1991; 20: 193-195.

13. Summerfield MJ, White PS: Ventilation tube insertion using topical anaesthesia in children. J Laryngol Otol 1992; 106: 427-428.

14. Kaddour HS: Myringoplasty under local anaesthesia: day case surgery. Clin Otolaryngol 1992; 17: 567-568.

15. Premachandra DJ: Use of EMLA cream as an analgesic in the management of painful otitis externa. J Laryngol Otol 1990; 104: 887-888.

16. El-Kholy A: Manipulation of the fractured nose using topical local anesthesia. J Laryngol Otol 1989; 103: 580-581.

17. Anniko M, Schmidt SH: The ototoxic potential of EMLA. Acta Otolaryngol (Stockh) 1988; 105: 255-265.

18. Anniko M, Hellstrom S, Schmidt SH, Spandow O: Toxic effects on inner ear of noxious agents passing through the round window membrane. Acta Otolaryngol (Stockh) Suppl 1988; 457: 49-56.

19. Schmidt SH, Hellstrom S, Anniko M: Effects of topical anesthesia on eardrum and inner ear. In: Recent Advances in Otitis Media. Lim DJL, Bluestone CD, Klein JO, Nelson JD, eds. BC Decker, Toronto: 1988; 413-416.

15

The Role of EMLA Cream in Split Skin Harvesting

Lennart Ohlsén

Uppsala University
Uppsala, Sweden

I. INTRODUCTION

The harvesting of split skin grafts for plastic surgery is a painful procedure that in the past has often required the use of general anesthesia, with its associated expense and potential risks. Anesthesia induced by injection of local anesthetics has been limited to small areas of skin, because the infiltration of anesthetics over large areas would be too painful. The development of topically applied EMLA® cream provided the possibility for painless induction of effective local anesthesia of the skin, which is of great potential in harvesting split skin grafts.

This chapter reviews studies designed to determine the safety and efficacy of EMLA cream in this indication, and discusses factors affecting them.

II. CLINICAL STUDIES

A. Study 1

Epicutaneous application of EMLA cream for cutting split skin grafts was first reported in 1985 by Ohlsén et al. [1] in a study involving 146 patients. The method used, in which EMLA cream (30 g/100 cm^2) was applied for about 2 hours under an occlusive dressing and elastic bandage, is described in Figures 1a to 1f. Split skin harvesting was carried out using standard procedures, and patients rated the pain experienced on a 4-point scale.

Analgesia was sufficient to permit removal of split skin grafts that included at least 50 to 75% of the thickness of the dermis. No pain (only the pressure of the dermatome) was experienced by 65% of the patients, and a further 19% mentioned only slight discomfort (Figure 2); no objection was made during cutting of the graft. Pain was described as moderate by 14% of patients, but only three patients (2%) described the pain as being severe and required additional analgesia. This was supplied by infiltration, which was likely to have been less painful than normal because the area was already partially anesthetized. No correlation was detected between the degree of pain experienced and whether premedication was provided.

The skin depth of sensory and pain thresholds depends on the application time of EMLA cream (see Chapter 2). In a study by Bjerring and Arendt-Nielsen [2], EMLA cream provided analgesia to a depth of 5 mm after application to intact skin for 120 minutes (Figure 3). The thickness of skin grafts in the study of Ohlsén [1] never exceeded 0.53 mm, and pain during the procedure was not correlated to the thickness of the graft, although a correlation was noted between the efficacy of EMLA cream and its application time (Figures 4, 5).

Ohlsén [1] noted a difference between men and women in the amount of pain reported. Male patients complained of insufficient analgesia more often than females (moderate to severe pain reported

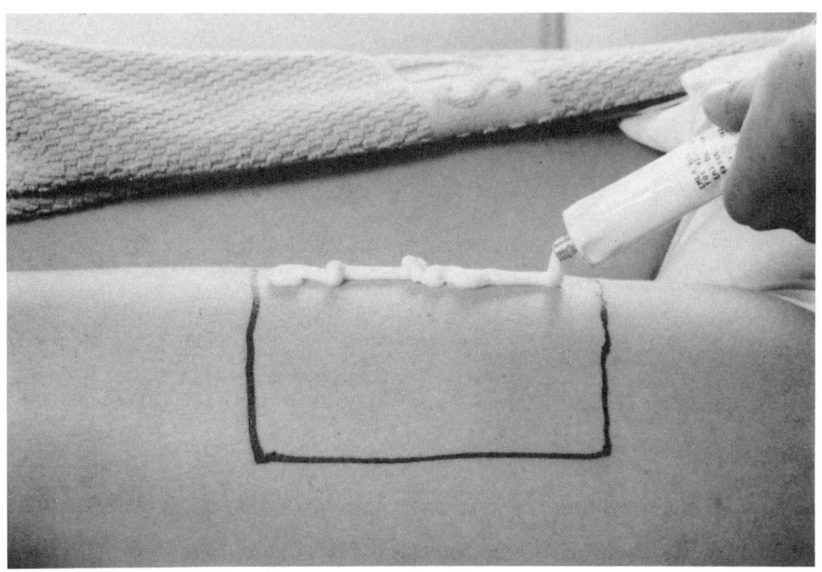

Figure 1a After the donor site has been marked, EMLA cream is applied to the skin.

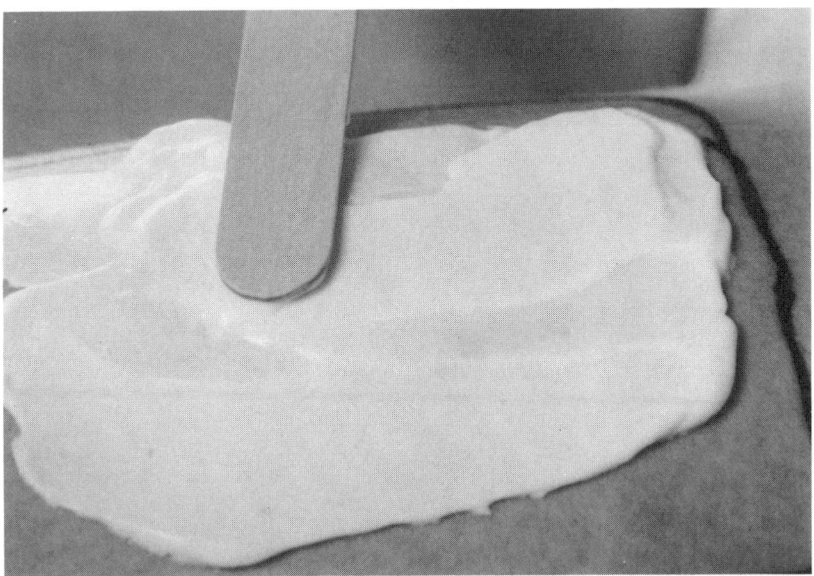

Figure 1b EMLA cream is applied in a thick layer covering the marked area.

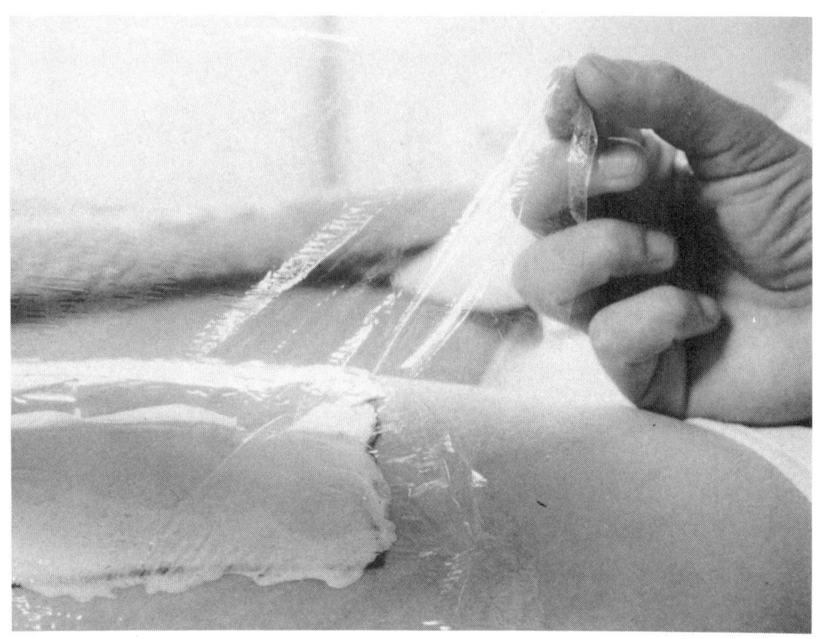

Figure 1c The cream is then covered with thin plastic foil.

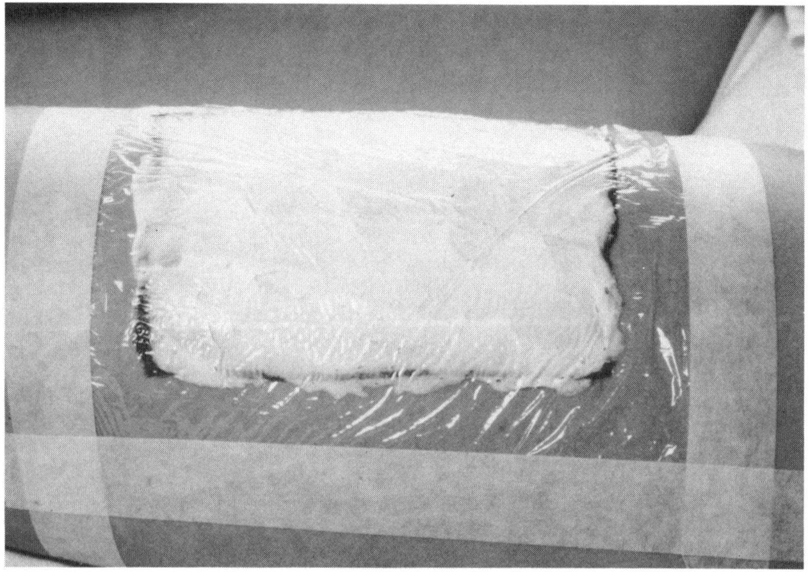

Figure 1d The plastic foil is taped to the skin.

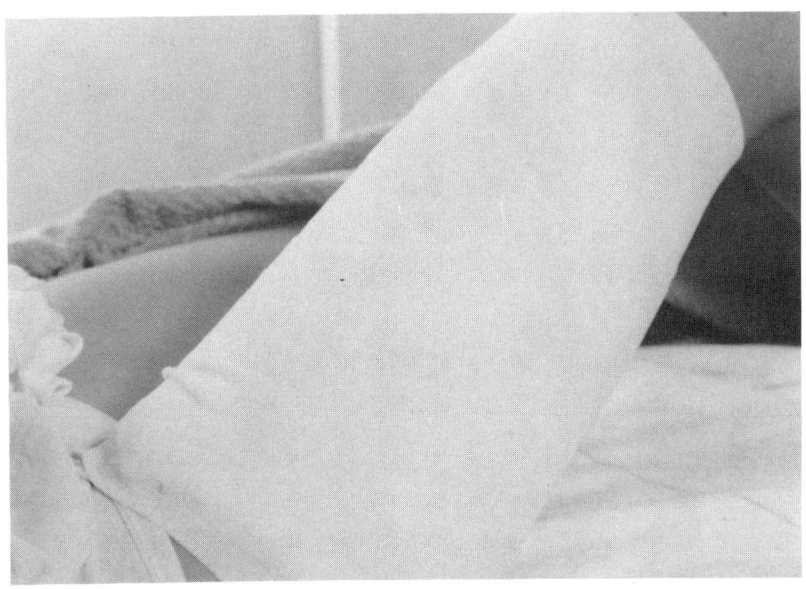

Figure 1e An elastic bandage is used to apply a slight compression.

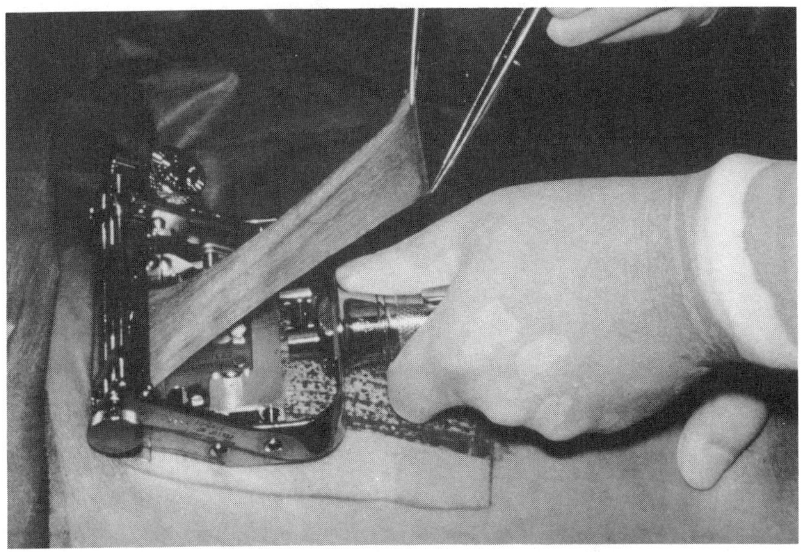

Figure 1f After an application time of 2 hours, the area is anesthetized and the split skin graft can be cut.

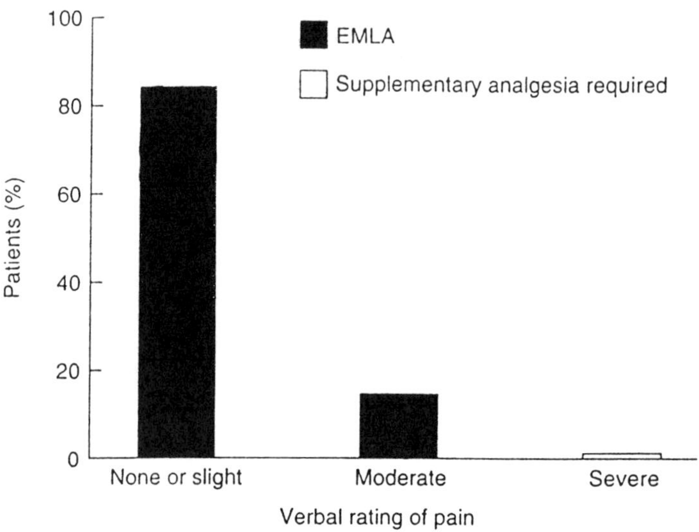

Figure 2 Verbal rating of pain in 146 patients when cutting split skin grafts in EMLA analgesia with a minimum application time of 2 hours. 143 patients did not require additional anesthesia.

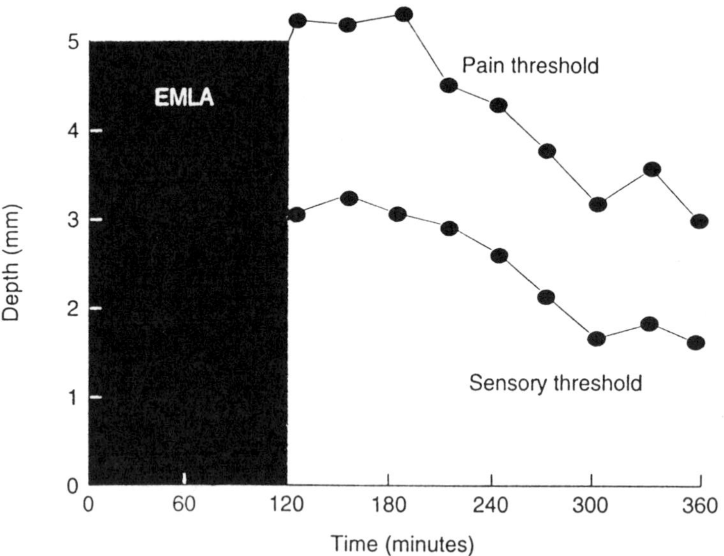

Figure 3 After application to intact skin for 2 hours, EMLA provides analgesia to a depth of 5 mm. The depth of sensory and pain thresholds were determined for up to 4 hours after application of 5 g EMLA to a skin area of 12 cm^2.

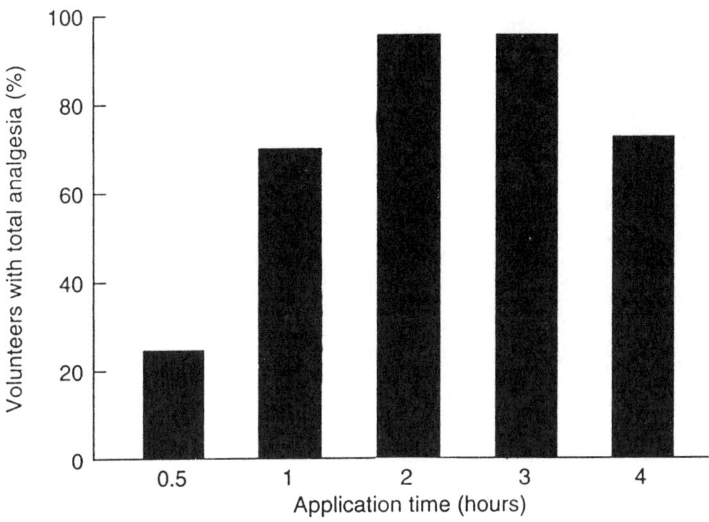

Figure 4 Dermal analgesia achieved with EMLA after different application times. Pinprick testing after application of 1 g EMLA to a skin area of 10 cm^2.

by 17% and 14%, respectively), in spite of a higher proportion of the men having received premedication. The difference was not thought to be due to differences in EMLA cream application time (the cream was applied for at least 3 hours in 40% of the men and 52% of the women), but may have resulted from differences in the choice of donor site in male and female patients (Figure 6).

Local effects included pallor (62 patients), erythema (42 patients) edema (14 patients) and mild, transient irritation (six patients). Blood levels of lidocaine and prilocaine, measured in 106 patients, did not exceed 1,100 ng/ml and 200 ng/ml, respectively.

B. Study 2

Lähteenmäki et al. [3] also described the use of EMLA cream in 1985, at the T. S. Society of Plastic Surgeons meeting in Finland. Of 26 operations for split skin harvesting, 23 were reported to have been

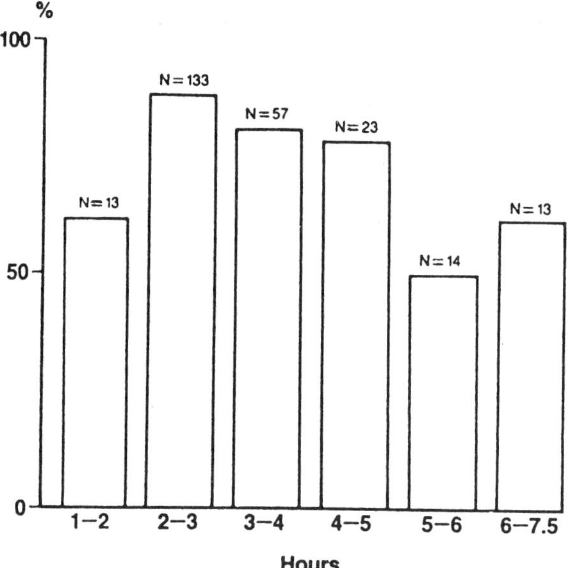

Figure 5 Relative frequency of no or slight pain compared to moderate or severe pain during cutting of split skin grafts in relation to application time of EMLA cream. Pooled data from 253 patients. Optimal dermal analgesia is achieved after application of EMLA for more than 2 hours and less than 5 hours.

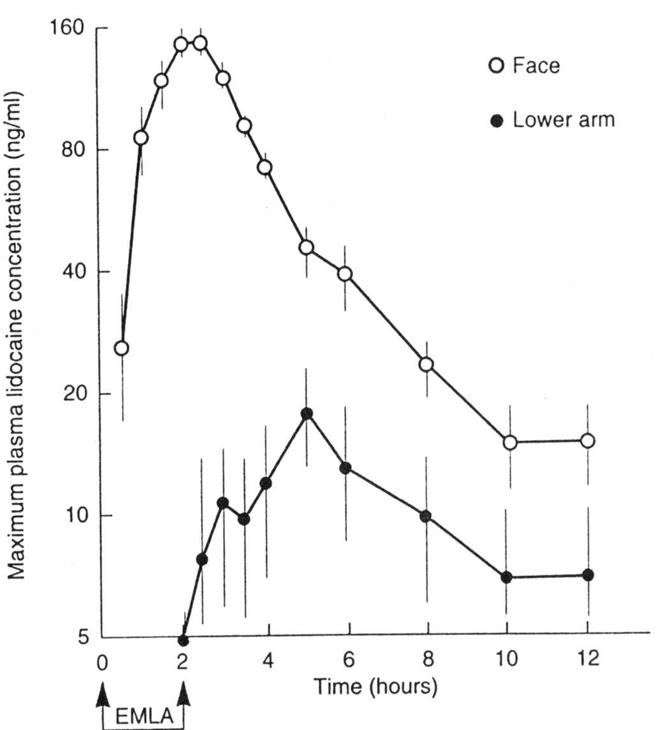

Figure 6 After 10 g of EMLA has been applied for 2 hours to a skin area of 100 cm^2, the maximum plasma concentration of lidocaine is reached after 2 hours when applied to the face but not until after 5 hours when applied to the forearm.

performed without pain. An additional four-center study by Lähteen-mäki was reported in 1988 [4]. The efficacy of two doses of EMLA cream, 30 g or 60 g per 200 cm^2, applied for 2 to 5 hours, was compared. Patients rated the degree of pain experienced on a 4-point scale; 92% of patients in both groups reported no or slight pain. There was no statistical difference between the two groups, either in efficacy of the applied dose of EMLA cream or in the number and severity of local reactions experienced. The latter were mild and included pallor, redness, edema and a burning sensation.

C. Study 3

An open, parallel-group study comparing EMLA cream with lidocaine infiltration in 80 patients was carried out by Goodacre [5]. Unlike those in previous investigations, most of the patients in this study did not receive premedication. The EMLA and lidocaine groups of patients were well matched demographically, but the mean area of skin har-vested was greater in the EMLA group (122 cm^2 vs. 69 cm^2). Pain experienced during administration of the anesthetic and harvesting of the graft was rated using a visual analog scale (VAS) of 0 to 100 and a 4-point verbal rating scale.

The pain scores for lidocaine infiltration ranged from 13 to 89 and correlated with the volume of anesthetic administered; a pain score of zero was noted for administration of EMLA cream. The mean VAS pain score for graft cutting was 8 in the EMLA group and 11 in the lidocaine infiltration group. On the verbal rating scales, 27 of 37 assessable patients in the EMLA group rated the procedure as painless and eight rated the pain as "slight"; in the lidocaine group 20 out of 40 patients reported no pain and 17 reported slight pain. These differ-ences were not statistically significant. Local effects were similar in both groups and included pallor, pilar erection, erythema and tingling (Figure 7).

The authors concluded that the efficacy of EMLA cream was at least equal to that of lidocaine infiltration, and the painless adminis-tration allowed larger areas of skin to be anesthetized. EMLA cream was particularly useful in an outpatient setting, and could facilitate carrying out split skin harvesting as a day-care surgery procedure.

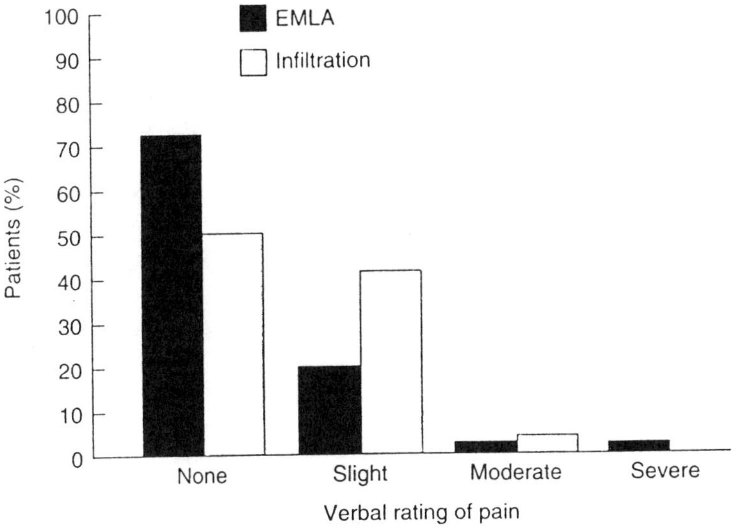

Figure 7 Patient's rating of pain measured on a verbal rating scale, experienced during harvesting of split skin grafts in analgesia obtained by EMLA or lidocaine infiltration.

D. Study 4

Strömbeck et al. [6] reported a study in which EMLA cream was applied for 1 to 8 hours. Of the 83 patients, 72 (87%) underwent split skin harvesting without any supplementary analgesia. Pain was rated as "none" or "slight" by 60 patients; 16 patients rated the pain experienced as "moderate" and six rated pain as "severe." The best analgesic effect was obtained with application times of less than 5 hours. No adverse influence on the viability of the graft or the healing of the donor site was noted. The authors reported that use of EMLA cream for harvesting split skin grafts is now routine at their clinic.

E. Other Studies

Bucyk et al. [7] evaluated the efficacy of EMLA cream during split skin harvesting on upper limbs and assessed the use of EMLA in combination with a 1.5% carbon dioxide lidocaine-induced brachial plexus block. One of 10 patients complained of pain during skin harvesting.

Cesany and Raska [8] compared three methods of local anesthesia for taking skin transplants: procaine injection, freezing with chloroethyl-kelene, and EMLA cream. Only one of 25 patients given EMLA anesthesia reported pain, and the authors favored EMLA cream as the optimal method of providing anesthesia.

Ohlsén et al. [9] used EMLA analgesia for harvesting split skin grafts concomitantly with debridement of ulcers. Only two of 22 patients reported moderate pain, and it was not necessary to administer additional analgesia.

III. FACTORS AFFECTING USE OF EMLA FOR SPLIT SKIN HARVESTING

A. Assessment of Pain

Clinical trials carried out to assess alleviation of pain are always liable to be affected by a "mental factor." The patient is aware that a new method of achieving analgesia is being tested and is thus more sensitive to the possibility of its failure. More recent experience in the use of EMLA cream in a setting where its use for cutting skin grafts is routine suggests that patients do not complain of any pain during the procedure [Ohlsén, unpublished observation].

It can be difficult for some patients to dissociate the sensation of vibration and pressure from the dermatome—which are experienced even with anesthesia—from feelings of pain. The application of EMLA cream, or any other epicutaneous anesthetic, induces a decrease or loss of perception of painful stimuli and suppresses the excitability of C receptors, but does not remove all sensory feelings. The sense of touch is decreased, but the pressure and vibration of the dermatome is always felt. Indeed, moving a hair in the anesthetized area can be felt [1,7], as can the pressure of a pin, although no pain from the pinprick is experienced. Pinprick tests should be avoided when assessing analgesia, as the sensations generated can be worrying to the patient [6]. Also to be avoided is warming the anesthetized area, for example, by washing the application area with warm water, because sensitivity to warmth (but not cold) is increased [1].

B. Application Time and Dose

The efficacy of EMLA cream depends on the application time used. Pooled data from clinical studies involving a total of 253 patients suggest that, for harvesting split skin grafts, EMLA cream application times of 2 to 5 hours provide the most effective analgesia [4]. For application times outside this range, the frequency of adequate analgesia is lower. It should, however, be noted that for application times of less than 2 hours, improvement in analgesia continues after removal of the cream.

The stratum corneum appears to act as a reservoir for supply of EMLA to underlying tissue [10]. Provided that the applied dose of EMLA cream is sufficient to maintain a full-stratum corneum reservoir, there is no reason to expect dose dependency in the efficacy of EMLA cream. One study specifically designed to investigate dose dependency [4] showed that there was no correlation between dose and efficacy of EMLA cream when application times of over 3 hours were used. Other studies, however, have noted that the analgesic effect of EMLA cream appeared to be dose-related [11–13].

The application time necessary for split skin harvesting is longer than that required for other indications. For example, 60 minutes is the recommended application time for venipuncture (see Chapter 3) and analgesia has been demonstrated after only 15 minutes [12,14–16]. The longer application time necessitates the introduction of measures to ensure that the cream is well homogenized while it remains in contact with the skin. Over time, the anesthetic oil droplets next to the skin become depleted, and it has been shown that if the concentration of EMLA falls below 0.8%, no oil droplets are present [17]. This could cause a decrease in drug penetration into the skin. Therefore, during the long application times for split skin harvesting, the occlusive dressing and bandage covering the cream should be massaged at least hourly to ensure redistribution of the oil droplets within the EMLA cream.

The duration of application is important to ensure adequate analgesia not only during cutting of split skin grafts but also postoperatively. The duration of analgesia after a 1-hour application of EMLA cream is between 1 and 5 hours (depending on location) [12]. Following the cutting of skin grafts under EMLA anesthesia, the duration of analgesia has been reported to be several hours [1]. After the operation, patients complained about pain from the donor site less often than could be expected from prior experience with patients receiving general anesthesia.

C.   Success of Skin Grafts

None of the studies using EMLA cream for cutting split skin grafts [1,3–6,8,9] reported any difference in the bleeding time or healing time at the donor site, or healing at the grafted site, compared to grafts taken under general anesthesia. A postoperative histological investigation did not show any changes in the quality of skin graft following application of EMLA cream. Duhnér and Lewis [18] report that EMLA allows blood vessels within the skin to revert to normal tone, which would explain the lack of effect on bleeding time compared to general anesthesia. Local infiltration with lidocaine-adrenaline gives rise to less bleeding than EMLA cream, due to the vasoconstrictive properties of adrenaline.

D.   Local Reactions

The longer application times and larger skin areas that must be covered by EMLA cream for harvesting split skin grafts have led to studies investigating its safety for this indication. The mild local reactions that commonly occur with EMLA, such as pallor, erythema, burning and itching, have all been observed when the cream is used for this procedure.

Ohlsén [1] has suggested that the burning sensation could be caused by application of the alkaline cream (pH 9.4) to a newly shaved area, which may have suffered slight skin abrasions. The sensation is transient and fades as the local anesthetic is absorbed.

After removal of the EMLA cream, a local effect of pallor is common for application times of up to 2.5 hours [1,3,5–7,11–13,19]; however, after application times of 4 hours or more, this phenomenon is not seen. Pallor is succeeded by erythema for application times of over 2.5 hours [1,5,12,19]. The incidence and degree of erythema increases with increased application time [1,6], and it is thus more common in patients undergoing split skin graft harvesting. Both lidocaine and prilocaine have vasoconstrictor and vasodilator properties, depending on their concentration [20] (see Chapter 2). The lower concentrations of EMLA provided by shorter application times give rise to vasoconstriction and pallor. Longer application times provide higher concentrations, resulting in vasodilatation and erythema [19, 21]. Mild edema has also been observed on removal of the cream, but was considered clinically insignificant [1,4,22]. All these effects (pallor, erythema and edema) disappear within a few hours of removal of the cream.

E. Systemic Effects

Systemic absorption of lidocaine and prilocaine following epicutaneous application is very low (Figure 8) and the technique is not associated with any toxic effects [1,7–9,11]. The largest application area reported to date is 1,296 cm^2, which gave rise to maximum blood concentrations of 1.1 µg/ml for lidocaine and 0.2 µg/ml for prilocaine [1]. These values can be compared with those for lidocaine following

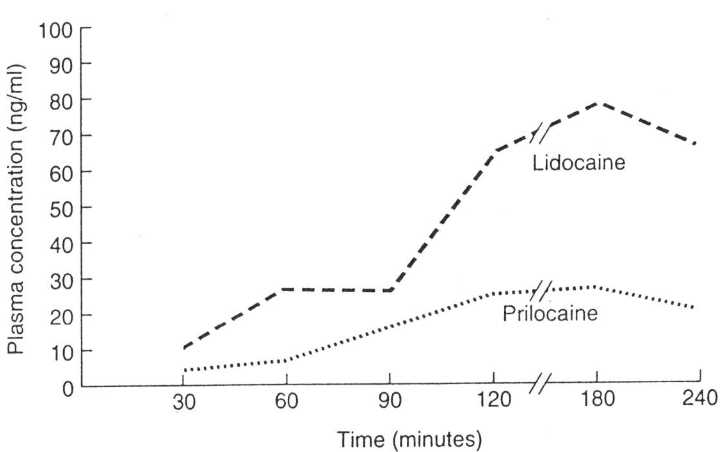

Figure 8 The plasma concentrations measured after application of 20 g EMLA cream for 60 minutes to a skin area of 300 cm^2.

brachial plexus blockade (peak blood level of 2.5 µg/ml for a 400 mg dose) or prilocaine following intercostal nerve blockade (mean blood concentration of 4.5 µg/ml for a 400 mg dose) [20]. Plasma concentrations of lidocaine and prilocaine were measured following the simultaneous use of EMLA cream at both a donor site for split skin harvesting (application time 250 minutes) and a leg ulcer site undergoing debridement (application time 30 minutes) [9]. Maximum levels, noted 35 minutes after removal of the cream, were 1.2 µg/ml (lidocaine) and 0.4 µg/ml (prilocaine).

Early signs of toxicity are only seen with lidocaine and prilocaine at plasma concentrations above 5 µg/ml. Between 5 and 10 µg/ml, the likelihood of severe CNS toxicity progressively increases. The plasma concentrations obtained with epicutaneous application of EMLA cream for split skin harvesting are thus well below toxic levels. However, as prilocaine metabolites can give rise to methemoglobinemia in young infants (see Chapter 2), the recommended dose and application time should be strictly adhered to in such patients.

IV. CONCLUSION

The efficacy of EMLA cream has been shown to be equal to that of conventional infiltration as a local anesthetic for harvesting split skin grafts. Unlike infiltration, administration of topical EMLA cream is virtually pain-free. In addition, EMLA cream is well tolerated, with only transient and clinically insignificant local reactions being observed. It carries less risk of systemic side effects than if a donor area of similar size were to be infiltrated by a local anesthetic. Thus EMLA cream provides the opportunity to anesthetize large areas without concerns of toxicity or infliction of pain, and can therefore emulate more closely the situation experienced when using general anesthesia.

The requirement for a 2- to 5-hour waiting period can usually be incorporated into the operation schedule, and patients willingly accept the wait if potentially painful injections can be avoided as a result. Use of EMLA cream can facilitate performing split skin harvesting as a simple, pain-free outpatient procedure, which has cost and time advantages that are important in the current climate of financial constraint.

REFERENCES

1. Ohlsén L, Englesson S, Evers H: An anaesthetic lidocaine/prilocaine cream (EMLA) for epicutaneous application tested for cutting split skin grafts. Scand J Plast Reconstr Surg 1985; 19: 210-209.

2. Bjerring P, Arendt-Nielsen L: Depth and duration of skin analgesia to needle insertion after topical application of EMLA cream. Br J Anaesth 1990; 64: 173-177.

3. Lähteenmäki T, Waris T, Asko-Seljavaara S, Sundell B: Topical anaesthesia for harvesting of split skin grafts by a eutectic lidocaine-prilocaine cream (EMLA 5%). A clinical study. TS Soc Plast Surg Congr. Espoo, Finland, June 1985. Abstract 33.

4. Lähteenmäki T, Lillieborg S, Ohlsén L, Olenius M, Strömbeck J-O: Topical analgesia for the cutting of split-skin grafts: A multicenter comparison to two doses of lidocaine/prilocaine cream. Plast Reconstr Surg 1988; 82: 458-462.

5. Goodacre TEE, Sanders R, Watt DA, Stoker M: Split skin grafting using topical local anaesthesia (EMLA): A comparison with infiltrated anaesthesia. Br J Plast Surg 1988; 41: 533-538.

6. Strömbeck JO, Uggla M, Lillieborg S: Percutaneous anaesthesia with a lidocaine-prilocaine cream (EMLA) for cutting split-skin grafts. Eur J Plast Surg 1988; 11: 49.

7. Bucyk B, Carle HL, LeGatt D, Finegan B: Evaluation of EMLA in providing split skin thickness skin graft donor site analgesia. Can J Anaesth 1988; Suppl 35.

8. Cesany P, Raska D: Skin graft harvesting under local anaesthesia. Acta Chir Plast 1990; 32: 11-15.

9. Ohlsén L, Grafford K, Evers H: EMLA cream as topical anaesthetic for ulcer debridement and simultaneous split skin grafting. Eur J Plast Surg 1993. Submitted.

10. Rougier A, Dupuis D, Lotte C, Roguet R: The measurement of the stratum corneum reservoir. A predictive method in vivo percutaneous absorption studies: Influence of application time. J Invest Dermatol 1985; 84: 66-68.

11. Evers H, von Dardel O, Juhlin L, Ohlsén L, Vinnars E: Dermal effects of compositions based on the eutectic mixture of lignocaine and prilocaine (EMLA). Studies in volunteers. Br J Anaesth 1985; 57: 997.

12. Juhlin L, Evers H: EMLA: a new topical anaesthetic. Adv Dermatol 1990; 5: 75-92.

13. Juhlin L, Evers H, Broberg F: A lidocaine-prilocaine cream for superficial skin surgery and painful lesions. Acta Derm Venereol (Stockh) 1980; 60: 544-546.

14. Arendt-Nielsen L, Bjerring P: The effect of topically applied anaesthetics (EMLA cream) on thresholds to thermode and argon laser stimulation. Acta Anaesthesiol Scand 1989; 33: 469-473.

15. Ehrenström-Reiz G, Reiz S, Stockholm O: Topical anaesthesia with EMLA, a new lidocaine-prilocaine cream and the Cusum technique for detection of minimal application time. Acta Anaesthesiol Scand 1983; 27: 510-512.

16. Maddi R, Concepcion M, Horrow J, Mark J, Covino B, Murray E: Evaluation of EMLA as a topical anesthetic. Rec Anesth 1985; 10: 39.

17. Brodin A, Nyquist-Mayer A, Vadsten T, Forslund B, Broberg F: Phase diagram and aqueous solubility of the lidocaine-prilocaine binary system. J Pharm Sci 1984; 73: 481-484.

18. Dhuner K-G, Lewis DH: Effect of local anaesthetics and vasoconstrictors upon regional blood flow. Acta Anaesth Scand 1966 (Suppl 23); 347.

19. Bjerring P, Andersen PH, Arendt-Nielson L: Vascular response of human skin after analgesia with EMLA cream. Br J Anaesth 1989; 63: 655-660.

20. Covino B, Vasallo H: Local anaesthetics. In: Mechanisms of Action and Clinical Use. Grune & Stratton, New York: 1976.

21. Willatts DG, Reynolds F: Comparison of the vasoactivity of amide and ester local anaesthetics. Br J Anaesth 1985; 57: 1006-1011.

22. Hallen B, Carlsson P, Uppfeldt A. Clinical study of lignocaine-prilocaine cream to relief the pain of venepuncture. Br J Anaesth 1985; 57: 326-328.

16

A Study Investigating the Use of EMLA for Chronic Subcutaneous Drug Administration

Matitiahu Berkovitch

Assaf Harofe Hospital
Tzrifim, Israel

Susan Davis Lethbridge, Judy Donsky, Richard Hackman, Graham Sher, Gideon Koren, and Nancy Olivieri

The Hospital for Sick Children
Toronto, Ontario, Canada

Doreen Matsui

Children's Hospital of Western Ontario
London, Ontario, Canada

I. INTRODUCTION

The efficacy of EMLA® cream in alleviating the pain associated with many medical procedures that are performed once or periodically has been frequently documented [1]. However, there are many patients suffering from chronic illnesses, such as diabetes or thalassaemia, who require repeated painful procedures on a daily basis, and these patients have, to date, been largely ignored in studies with EMLA cream. The pain and inconvenience associated with required procedures such as injections and infusion are common reasons for emerging noncompliance among such patients, even with life-saving therapies [2].

For example, nightly therapy with subcutaneous deferoxamine (DFO), initiated in most developed countries in the 1970s for the treatment of iron overload, has been demonstrated to improve liver function [3,4], stabilize hepatic fibrosis [3], prevent iron-related cardiac [5] and gonadal [6] dysfunction, and extend survival [7] in transfusion-dependent thalassaemia patients. While the efficacy and safety of DFO are not debated, the difficulties associated with prolonged parenteral infusion of the drug on a nightly basis—a cumbersome, often irritating mode of administration—cannot be underestimated. The effectiveness of DFO is reduced in many adolescents and young adults, for whom the regimen represents a tremendous disruption of lifestyle [8] and in whom compliance is often erratic [2]. This is a major obstacle in the prevention of iron-related disease in developed countries, and survival could be extended significantly if compliance with chelation therapy could be improved [9].

It is acknowledged that compliance with therapy is reduced when the regimen is painful, complex, dependent on an alteration of a patient's lifestyle, inconvenient or expensive [10], as is the case with the use of parenteral DFO. However, since regular administration of iron-chelating therapy in transfusion-dependent patients is required for survival, good long-term compliance must be achieved. It may be possible to improve acceptance of the therapy if any pain associated with needle insertion and subcutaneous infusion of DFO is alleviated.

This chapter describes a recent study of the use of EMLA cream in patients with transfusion-dependent β-thalassaemia (HBT); the efficacy of EMLA cream in alleviating pain associated with needle insertion was investigated. The study was conducted in two parts:

1. An open study in which patients were asked to compare the pain experienced on needle insertion with EMLA cream to that exper-

ienced when the needle was inserted in the normal manner without analgesia

2. A double-blind, placebo-controlled, cross-over study in which EMLA and placebo creams were applied randomly on consecutive evenings

II. OPEN STUDY

EMLA cream was utilized in 12 children (six boys and six girls; mean age 11.8 ± 2.5 years) with transfusion-dependent HBT whose therapy included 12-hour subcutaneous infusions of DFO, 5 to 7 nights a week. Each patient was instructed to apply, 1 hour prior to the initiation of infusion, a thick layer of EMLA cream (approximately 1.5 g per 7 cm^2), covered by an occlusive dressing (Tegaderm®), over the planned site of needle insertion. Following insertion of the transfusion needle, the patients were asked to rate the degree of pain on a 100 mm visual analog scale (VAS) with 0 mm representing "no pain" and 100 mm representing "the worst pain you can think of." The following evening the patients were instructed to insert the needle in the routine way, without the use of EMLA cream, and to mark the degree of pain on an identical VAS.

Nine of the 12 subjects reported some degree of pain associated with needle insertion during the routine procedure without EMLA cream. These patients reported "no pain" when EMLA cream was used. In the remaining three patients, no pain was reported either with or without the use of EMLA cream. Pain as assessed by the VAS was significantly lower ($p = 0.005$) with EMLA cream than with no cream (1.5 ± 2.2 mm vs. 34.8 ± 33.5 mm, respectively).

III. BLINDED STUDY

A second group of 10 subjects (five males and five females; mean age 18.3 ± 5.7, mean duration of treatment 11.5 ± 4.5 years), were randomly assigned to apply, in the manner described above, either EMLA or placebo cream (1.5 g) to the proposed site of needle insertion. The following evening the other cream was used. Both creams were identical in appearance and odor. Patients were instructed to rate the pain of needle insertion using the previously described VAS.

The degree of pain experienced was significantly less with EMLA cream (5.7 ± 8.2 mm) than with placebo cream (27.0 ± 22.8 mm) ($p = 0.01$). Three patients reported "no pain" upon insertion of the needle when EMLA cream was used, despite experiencing pain with the placebo cream. Two patients reported no pain on needle insertion with either placebo or EMLA cream.

No adverse effects were reported with the use of either EMLA or placebo cream.

IV. DISCUSSION

Olivieri et al. [2] reported a dramatic decrease in compliance with the regimen of subcutaneous DFO in patients between 10 and 20 years old. This observation was made at a time when DFO-related neurotoxicity was under investigation [11], and large amounts of DFO and supplies were being recalled. It has been noted that most physicians overestimate their patients' compliance [12], and a generally low rate of adherence to chronic medical regimes must be expected. Specific measures must therefore be adopted to increase patient compliance [13].

The majority of older children in the study described here judged the pain of needle insertion to be nullified by the cream. However, in five of the HBT patients, needle-insertion pain was rated as zero even without EMLA analgesia, and it could be argued that these children, being used to such pain, may not benefit from the local anesthetics. The alleviation of pain associated with subcutaneous needle insertion shown in HBT patients agrees with the results of Taddio et al. [14] (see Chapter 8), who demonstrated the efficacy of EMLA cream in alleviating the pain of subcutaneous injection in volunteers and patients during vaccination. It is likely that the pain experienced with nightly subcutaneous infusions of DFO consists of skin penetration and a second, deeper pain. The studies with vaccination indicated that EMLA cream is effective in reducing not only the superficial pain but also some of the deeper pain, which may be another factor in increasing compliance in thalassaemia.

To be effective in thalassaemia patients, EMLA cream would need to be applied nightly. This requirement raises the need for studies addressing the safety of chronic use of EMLA cream, in particular the risk of development of methemoglobinemia. It is extremely unlikely that adolescent or adult patients would suffer from dose-dependent toxicity from either lidocaine or prilocaine following nightly use of the cream. The issue of sensitization of patients and the emergence of allergic reactions should be kept in mind, however, because such reactions can occur with other modes of application of local anesthetics.

V. CONCLUSION

In the future, it will be pivotal to investigate specific determinants leading to impaired compliance with DFO in adolescents with thalassaemia. If such analysis reveals that the pain associated with the nightly subcutaneous infusion of the drug is a major source of concern, discomfort and fear for the youngsters, the results of these studies show that EMLA analgesia may be helpful and the cream should be made available to such children.

During the next few years, the medical community should explore the use of EMLA cream for pediatric and adult patients who have to endure procedure-related pain on a daily basis. It is likely that EMLA cream will have a major impact on the quality of life of these patients, and hence on their compliance with pharmacotherapy.

REFERENCES

1. Koren G: Use of the eutectic mixture of local anesthetics in young children for procedure-related pain. J Pediatr 1993; 122 (suppl): 530-535.
2. Olivieri NG, McGee A, Liu P, Koren G, Freedman MH, Benson L: Cardiac disease free survival in patients with thalassemia major treated with subcutaneous deferoxamine: an update of the Toronto cohort. Ann NY Acad Sci 1990; 612: 585.

3. Barry M, Flynn D, Letsky E, Risdon RA: Long-term chelation therapy in thalassemia major: effect of liver iron concentration, liver histology and clinical progress. Br Med J 1974; 2: 16-24.

4. Cohen AR, Martin M, Schwartz E: Depletion of excessive liver iron stores with desferrioxamine. Br J Haematol 1984; 58: 369-373.

5. Wolfe LC, Olivieri NF, Sallan D et al.: Prevention of cardiac disease with subcutaneous desferrioxamine in patients with thalassemia major. N Engl J Med 1985; 312: 1600-1603.

6. Bronspiegel-Weintrob N, Olivieri NF, Tyler BJ et al.: Effect of age at the start of iron chelation therapy on gonadal function in beta thalassemia major. N Engl J Med 1990; 323: 713-719.

7. Zurlo MR, De Stefano P, Borgna-Pignatti C et al.: Survival and causes of death in thalassemia major. Lancet 1989; ii: 27-30.

8. Cohen AR: Iron overload in the pediatric patient. Hematol Oncol Clin North Am 1987; 1: 521-544.

9. Fosburg M, Nathan DG: Treatment of Cooley's anemia. Blood 1990; 76: 435-444.

10. Haynes RB. Introduction. In: Compliance in Health Care. Haynes RB, Sackett DL (eds). Baltimore: Johns Hopkins University Press, 1979; 1-7.

11. Olivieri NF, Buncic JR, Chew E et al.: Visual and auditory neurotoxicity in patients receiving deferoxamine infusions. N Engl J Med 1986; 314: 869-873.

12. Caron HS, Roth HP: Patients' cooperation with a medical regimen. J Am Med Assoc 1968; 203: 922-926.

13. Inui JF, Yourtee EF, Williamson JW: Improved outcomes in hypertension after physician tutorials. Ann Intern Med 1976; 84: 649-651.

14. Taddio A, Robieux I, Koren G: Effect of lidocaine-prilocaine cream on pain from subcutaneous injection. Clin Pharm 1992; 11: 347-349.

17

The Impact of EMLA on the Ethics of Pediatric Research

Gideon Koren

The Hospital for Sick Children
Toronto, Ontario, Canada

I. INTRODUCTION

The involvement of children in medical research is necessary in order to advance knowledge on the normal and abnormal development of children, to determine the nature of their illnesses, and for the development of appropriate new therapies.

Collection of the data needed for such research very often calls for sampling of body fluids. Blood is by far the most common type of sample required, but access to blood is regarded by ethicists and clinicians alike as involving "invasive" procedures. When research is done with consenting adults, their affirmation acknowledges that they have considered the risk-benefit ratio of such procedures. Children cannot legally consent, and therefore the burden of making appropriate decisions lies with the legal guardians, with the research ethics committee and, indeed, with the community in its larger sense.

The construct of risk-benefit ratio in pediatric research is a constant struggle for research ethics committees worldwide. This last chapter illuminates some of the major considerations taken into account in most Western countries to date, and discusses the impact that painless needle insertion, possible with the use of EMLA® cream, could have on the assessment of risk-benefit ratios in research.

II. RISK CATEGORIES

Any potential risk involved in pediatric research should be measured against the "baseline" risk for the particular child. This baseline risk is defined in the United States and Canada as "minimal" and in the United Kingdom as "negligible": it has been described by the U.S. Department of Health and Human Services (DHHS) regulations as that "ordinarily encountered in daily life or during the performance of routine physical or psychological examinations or tests" [1].

The DHHS has defined the three categories of risk described below; these are also accepted in the United Kingdom [2], although with slightly different terms.

A. Minimal Risk (With or Without Benefit to the Child)

Studies involving minimal risk may include, for example, observation of a child's normal functions or the collection of routine clinical and laboratory data. Routine immunizations, modest changes in diet, obtaining blood or urine samples and developmental tests could all be categorized as involving minimal risk. Research ethics committees generally do not have problems in approving such protocols, assuming that scientific validity has been established and that informed consent and assent have been obtained.

B.   Minor Increase over Minimal Risk

It is generally accepted that in this category the risk of death is between 1 and 100 per million, of major complication 10 and 1000 per million, and of minor complication 1 and 100 per thousand.

In addition to proving the scientific validity of such a project and obtaining consent and assent, researchers have to ensure that the risk is justified by the anticipated benefits to the child, and that the anticipated benefit relative to potential risk is at least as favorable as that presented by available alternatives.

There are two categories of potential benefit that may be used to calculate the risk-benefit ratio:

1. The research presents the prospect of direct benefit to the studied child.
2. There is no prospect of direct benefit to the studied child, but the research is likely to yield general (and helpful) knowledge about the disorder or condition.

According to the DHHS, it is a prerequisite that the procedures experienced by the studied children be "reasonably commensurate with those inherent in their actual or expected medical, dental, psychological, social or educational situations." For example, the American Academy of Pediatrics finds it acceptable to ask a child whether he or she would be willing to undergo an additional bone marrow aspiration for research purposes, provided the child has had previous bone marrow aspirations or will need to have them during the course of treatment [3]. The demand for commensurability assumes that a child who has already experienced a procedure during the conduct of medical care has a level of knowledge that is appropriate for deciding whether to participate in research requiring that procedure.

An important prerequisite for the approval of studies in this category is that the knowledge anticipated from the study be of vital importance for understanding or ameliorating the child's disorder or condition. This demand is not requested in studies with only minimal risk, thus recognizing that the usefulness of the study data must counterbalance the higher risk, and reflecting a higher level of concern.

C. Risk Greater than Minor Increase over Minimal Risk

According to the DHHS, protocols in this category should be approved only if the local research ethics committee "finds that the research represents a reasonable opportunity to further the understanding, prevention or alleviation of a serious problem affecting the health and welfare of children." Such research carries a risk of death of more than 100 per million, of major complication greater than 1000 per million, and of minor complication greater than 100 per thousand. In the United States, the secretary of the appropriate governmental agency must approve research with such excessive risk, after consultation with a panel of experts.

III. RISK ANALYSIS

In most countries, the regulations allow the local research ethics committee to define a "minor increase over minimal risk." A basic problem with this definition is the difficulty in assessing the baseline risk associated with normal medical procedures (Table 1 [4–12]). The American Academy of Pediatrics submits that most publications accept venipuncture and intravenous infusions as posing "minimal risk" [3], and this approach, at least with respect to venipuncture, is also accepted in the United Kingdom [5].

Because the degree of risk involved in a variety of procedures varies with both the expertise of those performing them and the technology available locally, it is important for the research ethics committee to obtain information about the normal practices of the institution where the research is to be carried out.

In general, it is more simple to approve pediatric research with risk above minimal when direct benefit to the child is likely; when no such benefit is expected, the approval process may be more difficult. In fact, the Working Group convened by the British Institute of Medical Ethics agreed unanimously that it was not acceptable to subject children to even a minor increase over minimal risk in non-therapeutic research: "In other words, non therapeutic research on children, regardless of possible benefits, can only be undertaken ethically if the risks of the procedure are in the 'minimal' category" [5]. This approach is in sharp contrast to the views represented by the American regulations, and may introduce difficulties in conducting a variety of protocols in the United Kingdom that may be acceptable in the United States.

Examples of procedures falling into the "greater than minimal" risk category that have been approved at Yale University include bone marrow aspirations in children with leukemia, an additional spinal tap in adolescents who have already had at least one such procedure for a neurologic disorder, and administration of yohimbine to study the pathogenesis of neurologic disorder. The same research ethics committee rejected a request to perform left heart catheterization on children at risk for the development of cardiac hemosiderosis [12]. During 1990, the Research Ethics Committee at the Hospital for Sick Children in Toronto approved a protocol performing percutaneous liver biopsy in iron-overload adolescents treated with an experimental iron chelator, an additional bone marrow aspiration in children with aplastic anemia treated with an experimental growth factor, and additional intestinal biopsy for immunologically impaired children with chronic diarrhea treated with oral gamma globulins.

A major obstacle in assessing the magnitude of the risk is the frequent lack of valid baseline data. Even for procedures where such figures are available (Table 1), the data generally are based on a maximum of a few hundred cases, and the confidence intervals remain very wide, so that the true risk for death or major complication can be easily placed in more than one risk category. Moreover, such risks as pain and discomfort are not commonly measured in a quantitative manner. Even when they are measured, it is impossible to combine such data with those of other risk factors that are usually measured in different "units."

More complex, numerical methods of risk-benefit analysis have been suggested as an alternative to personal assessment; however, they require far more background data and hypothetical assumptions are necessary. In one such method, Rosser and King have employed a graded score of total disutility or utility of a particular project [13]. It is not likely that these methods will be introduced for routine assessment of research protocols in pediatrics, as they are cumbersome, complicated and stem from assumptions that will have to be validated in pediatric patients. A common practical approach used

Table 1 Risk Reported for a Selected Group of Procedures

Procedure	Risk
Peripheral arterial puncture	19 per 1000 for major complication (major bruising, aneurysm in site); 390 per 1000 minor complications
Lumbar puncture	Meningitis secondary to puncture 132 per 1000 in neonate: 47% failure rate; some risk of meningitis secondary to puncture
Insertion of nasogastric tube	Peptic esophagitis with long-term intubation; major complication less than 10 per million
Small intestine biopsy (Crosby capsule)	Bleeding: 1.4/1000
Rigid sigmoidoscopy	Fatality risk of 100 per million due to risk of sedation
Sedation	Fatality risk of 100 per million
Percutaneous liver biopsy (with Menghini needle)	Death risk of 200 per million
Bromsulphophthalein test	Anaphylaxis: 6 per million; death: 3 per million
Sulfonamide administration	Hypersensitivity syndrome: 1 per 1000; hemolytic anemia: 0.5 per 1000; agranulocytosis: 1 per 1000
Penicillin administration	Risk of anaphylaxis: 150–400 per million

Source: Based on Refs. 4–12.

by pediatric research ethics committees is for members to consider whether they would allow their own children to participate in such research [14]. However, it has been argued that children of clinical scientists are more likely to be enrolled into studies due to enhanced parental awareness, and thus this approach may not be valid [14].

Because of the increased complexity and sophistication of pediatric research, it is crucial for the research ethics committee to consult specialists in the field of the research protocol, not only during the scientific review but also for accurate estimation of risks and benefits. A survey of Canadian health professionals serving on pediatric research ethics committees showed that members needed authoritative advice in order to decide how many blood samples, if any, should be permitted for pharmacokinetic studies in neonates [15].

Much of the work of the research ethics committees remains intuitive, since, although the accepted categories of risk estimation yield a general framework for assessment of risk-benefit ratios, quantitative data are not available. Acknowledging this fact, ethical reviews must be conducted carefully, after evaluating all available information on potential risks and benefits.

IV. EMLA IN PEDIATRIC RESEARCH

As highlighted throughout this volume, EMLA is clearly very effective in minimizing or ameliorating the pain inflicted on children by needle insertion, including venipuncture and lumbar puncture. This breakthrough is likely to bring about substantial changes in the calculation of risk-benefit ratios in pediatric research necessitating such invasive procedures. Such changes are likely to be most important in cases where there is no direct benefit to the involved child (e.g. in pharmacokinetic studies) because, at present, research ethics committees tend to hesitate to inflict pain and anxiety on children under such circumstances.

In fact, many protocols call for venipunctures in cases in which control data are needed, such as age-dependent normal values of electrolytes, hormones, drugs, etc. These data are never directly beneficial to the participating child, and research ethics committees are reluctant to approve such research. EMLA, with its extremely effective ability to alleviate or even nullify pain associated with venipuncture, will therefore exert a positive impact on the pace of generation of crucial background knowledge in pediatric medicine.

In Toronto, the Research Ethics Committee at The Hospital for Sick Children advises scientists to use EMLA cream for all venipunctures. Although it is premature to conduct a formal assessment, it is my impression that studies involving venipuncture with "no direct benefit to the child" have been approved more readily since the introduction of EMLA.

Similarly, there is experimental evidence of the efficacy of EMLA to achieve analgesia in neonates following heel-prick procedures and circumcision [16]. After the necessary steps to prove the safety and efficacy of EMLA in infants younger than 3 months of age in relation to methemoglobin formation, it is likely that EMLA will be used for this age group. Thus, EMLA may change in a similar manner the risk-benefit ratio in many protocols involving preterm and/or sick neonates.

Potential problems in the design of study protocols involving EMLA include the local skin pallor associated with the cream and the need to wait 60 minutes between EMLA application and venipuncture. Although the pallor is mild from a toxicological standpoint, it is capable of unblinding a protocol dealing with EMLA vs. placebo and should be taken into account when designing the trial. The impact of a waiting period on routine clinical practice, and procedures to overcome any problems that may be encountered, are discussed in Chapter 5. For research, the waiting period should form part of the study design. In my view, investigators should always do everything possible to prevent pain associated with pediatric research, even if this means longer hours for the researchers or their assistants.

At present, venipuncture is defined by most authorities as a "minimal risk" category. The use of EMLA, which obviates pain associated with the procedure, may nullify its attendant risk altogether in many children. With more and more children experiencing minimal or no pain with EMLA, anticipatory fear conditioned by previous venipunctures is likely to be diminished or even disappear.

V. CONCLUSION

The introduction of EMLA is an important breakthrough in pediatric research. With more and more legal and ethical boundaries being imposed on pediatric scientists, it is reassuring to witness a novel pharmaceutical answer to the concerns regarding potential risks of research on children.

REFERENCES

1. US Department of Health and Human Services: Final regulation amending basic HHS policy for the protection of human research subjects. Federal Register 1981; 46: 16 (January 26): 8366-8388.

2. British Paediatric Association: Guidelines to aid ethical committees considering research involving children. Arch Dis Child 1980; 55: 75-77.

3. Lambert G: Institutional responsibilities in pediatric ethics: The American Academy of Pediatrics new guidelines. Presented at Ethics of Research at the Outset of Life, Hospital for Sick Children, Toronto, Jan 14–16, 1991.

4. Work Group XII of the National Institute of Arthritis, Metabolism and Digestive Diseases Evaluation Effort on the Future of Digestive Disease Research: Human experimentation in digestive disease research. Gastroenterology 1975; 69: 1165-1182.

5. Nicholson RH (Ed). Medical research with children: Ethics, law and practice. Oxford University Press, 1986.

6. Gillies IDS, Morgan M, Sykes MK, Brown AG, Jones NO: The nature and incidence of complication of peripheral arterial puncture. Anaesthesia 1979; 34: 506-509.

7. Teele DW, Sashefsky B, Bakusan T, Klein JO: Meningitis after lumbar puncture in children with bacteremia. N Engl J Med 1981; 305: 1079-1081.

8. Schreiner RL, Kleiman MB: Incidence and effect of traumatic lumbar puncture in the neonate. Dev Med Child Neural 1979; 21: 483-487.

9. Westaby D, MacDougall BRD, Williams R: Liver biopsy as a day-case procedure: selection and complications in 200 consecutive patients. Br Med J 1980; 281: 1331-1332.

10. Cooksley WGE: Anaphylaxis to bromosulfophthalein. Med J Aust 1971; 257-258.

11. Goodman GGA, Goodman LS, Rall TW, Murad F: The pharmacological basis of therapeutics. 7th edn. Macmillan, New York: 1987; 1134-1136.

12. Levine RJ: Children as research subjects. In: Kopelman LM, Mosko JC, Macmillan (Eds.) Children Health Care: Moral and Social Issues. New York: Kluwer Academic Publishers, 1989; 73-87.

13. Rosser R, Kind P: A scale of valuation of states of illness: is there a social consensus? Int J Epidemiol 1978; 7: 347-358.

14. Koren G, Pastuszak A: Medical research in infants and children in the eighties: Analysis of rejected protocols. Pediatr Res 1990; 27: 423-435.

15. Koren G, Litwack J, Biggard DW: Using infants in drug research when there is no direct benefit to them: A survey of Canadian health professionals serving in ethical committees. Can Med Assoc J 1988; 138: 899-902.

16. Fitzgerald M, Millard C, MacIntosh N: Cutaneous hypersensitivity following peripheral tissue damage in newborn infants and its reversal with topical anaesthesia pain. 1989; 39: 31-36.

Index